Dr. Ann's
10-Step Diet

Dr. Ann's
10-Step Diet

Ann Kulze, M.D.

Top Ten Wellness and Fitness

ISBN: 0974832804

Library of Congress Control Number: 2004101871

Submit all requests for reprinting to:
Greenleaf Book Group LLC
4425 Mopac South, Suite 600
Longhorn Building, 3rd Floor
Austin, TX 78735

Published in the United States by
Top Ten Wellness and Fitness
Charleston, SC

www.10stepdiet.com

Cover design by Francine Smith
Cover photo by Michael Balderas
Layout design by Francince Smith and Allison Pickett
Illustration by Allison Pickett
Index by Laura Shelly, Erin Nelsen, and Jacylyn Gardner

First Edition

To my father, Harry B. Gregorie, Jr., M.D.,
for his brilliant example as the compassionate
and gifted healer I will always aspire to emulate.

To my husband, John C. Kulze III, M.D.,
for his steadfast love and unfailing support,
which allow me to successfully balance passion for
my work with loving devotion to my family.

ACKNOWLEDGMENTS

I am eternally grateful to everyone whose help, support, and influence has made this book a reality: Meg La Borde and Nicole Hirsh of Greenleaf Book Group for their patience, keen editing skills, and dogged commitment to the highest standards; Alicia Reuter, my trusted and faithful assistant, for her invaluable research and technical skills, which made this project so much easier; Nancy Casey and Nancy Hendrickson of Copy with Velocity, whose writing skills contributed to the initial version of the book; and Kevin Graham, Chef of the Chattooga Club, for lending his culinary brilliance to this project.

A special thanks goes to my good friends at Ruby Tuesday for introducing and presenting "Dr. Ann" to millions of American diners interested in eating smarter and improving their health; my faithful friend, supporter, and business mentor, John M. Rivers, Jr., for his inspirational success with this plan and taking the critical first step that made this book possible; Anne Pope for her enthusiasm, encouragement, and assistance in spreading my wellness message to as many people as possible; and Larry Burtschy for his refreshing wit, insightful business advice, and financial support.

I offer my heartfelt appreciation to my children and biggest cheerleaders, Liz, Frazier, Jack, and Lucie, for allowing me to spend stolen family time writing this book and for providing me invaluable, "hands on" experience with food and nutrition as I strive to provide them proper nourishment; my mother Jane and siblings, Harry, Brian, Etta, Becky, Dicksie, and Jane, for their love and encouragement in my wellness endeavors; my good friends and fellow mothers, Monti, Elizabeth, Karen, and Sally, for providing their ears and helping hands in times of need and sharing their spirits with me; and Cathy, my loyal household assistant, whose hard work makes my work possible.

For making this book possible, I'd like to thank the innumerable scientists, physicians, and researchers whose intellect, hard work, and perseverance provided the spectacular body of solid and compelling science this book draws from; wellness trailblazers, Andrew Weil, M.D., and Walter Willett, M.D., for teaching and inspiring me to become a true wellness warrior myself through their extraordinary literary works and professional examples.

And finally, I'm especially indebted to the thousands of patients and clients who have entrusted their lives to my care and whose experiences imparted the knowledge and wisdom that compelled me to write this book.

TABLE OF CONTENTS

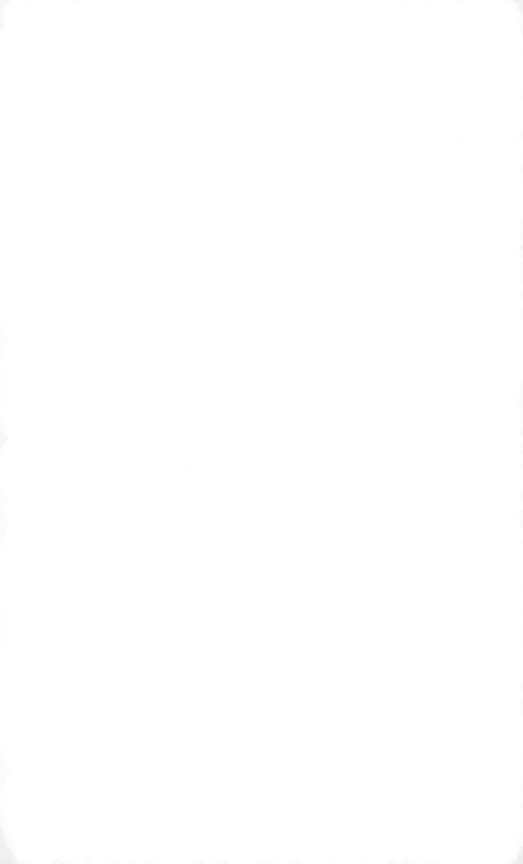

INTRODUCTION

THE JOURNEY BEGINS WITH JUST ONE STEP

I would like to introduce you to a new way of dieting—one that will make shedding those unwanted pounds easier, engage your mind, invigorate your body, lift your spirits, and still allow you to enjoy the delicious foods your body needs and loves.

The 10-Step Diet is an approach to weight loss that prides itself on taking the entirety of your wellness into account. It is grounded in the practice of eating well in order to live a healthier, longer life. And by following this diet, you will not only lose weight and look great, but you will also take major strides toward preventing most of the life-threatening chronic diseases experienced in this country. By making different choices about what you eat and how you live now, you can positively influence your health for the rest of your life. What's more, you will be able to enjoy those happy years with family and friends as the vibrant and healthy person you want to be.

In many ways, the 10-Step Diet is what I like to call a *lifestyle diet*, and it is probably rather different from diets and programs you've previously encountered. There are hundreds of diet books on the market already, and every year more are published. Each book claims to have uncovered the secret to weight loss, and while some of them do contain useful advice, very few of these books offer the nutritional information a dieter needs in order to lose weight *and* maintain it in the long run. Even fewer of these programs offer the insights that can help a dieter harness the profound, life-changing benefits the right foods provide.

It is no secret these days that a poor diet, loaded with sugar, red meat, and saturated fat can cause weight gain and provoke disease; but few people know that there are wonderful foods that can actually prevent disease *and* stimulate dramatic weight loss at the same time. You may not be aware of it, but the foods that will help you lose weight are the same foods that can ward off cancers, decrease the likelihood of dementia, and even prevent and reduce high cholesterol—and this is just the beginning.

If the 10-Step Diet has one mission, it is to help you benefit from these deliciously powerful foods. It is based on years of nutritional research and scientific investigation, and its goals are as easy to understand as the diet is to follow. This diet is not about losing weight through deprivation—only to put those pounds back on when your stamina breaks down—and it most certainly isn't about looking great at the *expense* of your health. Instead, it is a weight loss strategy that considers the entirety of your health to produce permanent, beneficial results inside and out.

This book, therefore, is designed to be the contemporary dieter's tool of empowerment. If there is anything my experience as a physician and wellness expert has shown me, Americans simply don't need any more new-fangled, rigid diets that are nearly impossible to incorporate into real life. What we need is the hard-won wisdom that has come from years of methodical, scientific study. Because of this notion, the 10-Step Diet encourages you to be as creative in your food choices as you want to be. I want you to enjoy what you eat, not merely for the tastes and pleasures of food, but also for the proven nourishment the *right* foods offer. I include sample recipes and meal suggestions, but keep in mind, the primary focus of this program is to impart the wisdom that will allow you to alter your favorite dishes to fit the guidelines established here and to discover and develop new recipes as well.

By equipping yourself with the nutritional facts, you will not only be capable of achieving your weight loss goals, but you will also be ready and able to make informed, lifelong dietary decisions on your own—and ultimately, this should be every dieter's goal. While many dieters just want to know *what* to eat, the people who have lasting success are those who understand *why* they should eat certain foods and avoid others. Once you have integrated the 10 Steps into your life and understand the rationale behind doing so, I know you won't need me any longer—in fact, the 10-Step Diet could very well be the last diet book you ever purchase.

The Birth of a Diet

Nutrition has always been one of my personal passions—you might even say it's somewhat of an obsession. The subject has intrigued me since my teens, and I determined early on that I would take that interest to college with me. After receiving a degree in Food Science and Human Nutrition from Clemson University, I heeded my father's sage advice to blend my passion with a medical education. Given that I hail from a long line of physicians, it wasn't surprising to anyone that I followed his suggestion. After postgraduate training in internal medicine, I took a position in a family medicine practice near my home in South Carolina.

But then something happened. Toward the end of 2001, I began to realize that my passion for food, diet, and nutrition—along with my interests in preventive medicine and teaching—were becoming more and more important to me; and unfortunately, my busy clinical practice precluded me from focusing on these things the way I wanted to. Simultaneously, I was alarmed to realize that my patients were not as healthy as they should have been—and more times than not, the health issues they were dealing with corresponded to their weight. Perhaps most startling, though, was knowing that these issues could have been avoided altogether. Those of my patients who *were* trying to lose weight were also losing heart; nothing seemed to work, they said, no matter which diet they tried.

The teacher in me was at a loss. At first, it was as though I had happened upon a child who had made his or her way through the first grade without learning how to read. How could my patients—and my fellow Americans, for that matter—have missed out on the basic strategies for healthy living? Upon reflection, however, it struck me that many of the people I spoke with were simply confused by the plethora of medical studies, FDA regulations, and fad diets that consistently fill the air waves and newspapers. And who could blame them? After all, how many families made the big switch from butter to margarine, only to find out later that most margarines are high in trans fat, one of the *worst* fats a person can ingest? How many others are still avoiding olive oil, nuts, and avocados—foods containing some of the *best* fats and nutrients a person can indulge in—because they have been told *all* fats are bad? We can say the same things for the recent blockbuster diets: low-fat, low-carb, high-protein, no-fat, no-carb, only protein. But which of these diets will help a person lose weight and maintain it? Which diet is the most practical? And most important, which diet is the *healthiest*?

Over the years, the American public has received numerous contradictory messages, and these messages have been confusing and exasperating for those of us who want to keep pace with the latest nutritional science. The good news is that these messages have been clarified in recent years, which is not to say that the medical community has reached the limit of nutritional research, but rather that the body of knowledge health practitioners and laymen can draw from is now far more complete and understandable.

This wakefulness has given rise to several good medical diets; however, many of these diets have been specifically fashioned to address concerns relating to heart disease and type 2 diabetes, often to the exclusion of other serious conditions that are also influenced by nutrition, such as cancer, Alzheimer's, and arthritis, to name just a few. Indeed, the medical community now knows that many of the illnesses and degenerative diseases our culture contends with are preventable through a variety of dietary and lifestyle modifications. We should pause to really consider this fact: just by eating certain foods and modestly changing our lifestyles, we can radically reduce our chances of becoming ill. It is a truly remarkable revelation, and one I want to help you take full advantage of.

So in 2002, with all these ideas and concerns top of mind, I decided to leave my clinical practice of fourteen years to begin a wellness consultation practice. My life has not been the same since.

I am not a "weight loss doctor," but rather a physician and a wellness expert. Though my recommendations consistently result in weight loss, my foremost goal has always been to provide each of my patients with a "whole person" wellness package unique to his or her individual situation. As a physician, I have watched too many of my patients struggle with their weight and the variety of diseases that can result from being overweight. As a wellness expert, however, I have been able to redirect the path my patients are going down by using a comprehensive approach to address their individual needs. But regardless of their specific concerns, the broad lessons are always the same: I teach my patients about the *right* fats, the *right* proteins, and the *right* carbohydrates. We discuss cooking techniques, how to identify the *wrong* foods from reading nutritional labels, and strategies to keep those dangerous items out of their shopping carts at the grocery store. I explain the almost drug-like properties of some of the most powerful foods available, such as blueberries, canned salmon, and broccoli. I preach the benefits of exercise and introduce them to other wellness ideas, including getting enough sleep, cultivating spirituality, and laughing often. It hasn't taken long to see the side-effects of this empowerment. Armed with straightforward and comprehensive information on nutritional and dietary strategies, my patients are losing weight easily, dramatically, and happily.

Since beginning my wellness practice, more and more clients have come to me specifically for weight loss guidance. It has been extremely rewarding to watch these people seize and understand the patterns of healthy eating and living that lead to sustainable weight loss. In the meantime, I have streamlined this information into the 10-Step Diet you now have in your hands. With the information here, I know that you can lose weight, look great, and most important, live a healthy, active life.

What to Expect from the 10 Steps

Weight loss in America is a complex matter, and like most complex matters, there is always more to the story than meets the eye.

We live in a culture where food plays a prominent role. It is virtually impossible to go anywhere in the country without seeing a billboard, TV ad, or magazine spread that is related to food. If you add that Americans are busier than ever before, you can begin to see the magnitude of the problem; at the end of a hard day of work, it's far easier to stop at McDonald's or order a pizza than it is to prepare a home-cooked meal.

Conversely, American culture bombards us with images of beauty and glamour that are contrived with airbrushes and digital manipulation, and these manufactured versions of beauty are nearly impossible to attain in real life. Between the sugary treats, the convenience of fast food, and the disparity between the image of beauty and the reality of it, it is no wonder so many Americans have thrown up their hands in dieting despair.

But that is only half of the story about weight loss. The other half of the story is that if you set your mind to it, you can do it. More importantly, losing weight the 10-Step way will set you on a path toward living a longer, healthier, and happier life. Of course, successful dieting requires you to do some work—you need to be informed, and you need to make smart, deliberate choices about what you eat and how often you exercise—but that doesn't mean you need to *suffer*. Indeed, as you will see throughout the 10 Step Diet, this program is all about *ending suffering*. After all, its primary aim is to help you lose weight that could, in the long run, be detrimental to your health.

What should you expect from the 10-Step Diet? It might be easier to start by telling you what you *shouldn't* expect. First, throw out the idea that dieting means eating strange foods or depriving yourself of great tastes. It is simply not true. If anything, this diet will introduce you to new, wonderful foods and the cooking techniques that will make them as flavorful as your palate desires.

Second, don't expect to be hungry. In fact, expect the opposite. One of the primary reasons diets "fail" is that hunger eventually overrides willpower. As the steps will teach you, the essential ingredient in weight loss is food. Eating the *right* foods will keep your body from triggering the hunger centers in your brain; and by reducing rapidly fluctuating blood sugar levels, along with decreasing the sensation of emptiness in your stomach, your weight loss efforts are sure to be far more successful than they would have been if you simply deprived yourself of the foods you crave and need.

Third, don't think you will be set apart from your family by virtue of eating well at the dinner table. As a working mother of four school-age children, I know there is nothing worse than watching your kids gobble down a plate of lasagna while you survey your bowl of steamed broccoli. Have no fear; this is a pragmatic plan, designed with your whole family's nutrition in mind. I have made sure that your entire family will like the foods included in this diet as much as you will. And of course, what is good for you is also good for the people you love.

Finally, while this diet does not require you to measure portions, count calories, or monitor carbohydrate and fat grams, it does encourage you to be mindful of the amounts and types of foods you are eating. It also requires you to do some work. When it comes to weight loss and your general health, exercise is non-negotiable. Unfortunately, too many diet books avoid stressing this fact for fear of being unpopular. And while I don't share this sentiment, I don't want to intimidate you either. Approached with the right mindset, exercise can be one of the most enjoyable aspects of your day; and furthermore, you will be surprised to see that even the smallest amount of physical exertion can have immense effects on your weight loss endeavor.

Now, how much weight can you expect to lose on the 10 Step Diet? This depends on how quickly you can incorporate all of the steps into your daily life. Part of the beauty of the 10 Step Diet is that it can be implemented at your own pace; but the sooner you integrate each step, the sooner you will accomplish your weight loss and wellness goals.

The 10-Step Diet is designed to take advantage of the proven, long-term success that comes with gradual weight loss over time. Solid weight loss science has consistently shown that the way to maintain weight loss is to lose weight in a gradual and steady manner over an extended period of time. Sudden and rapid weight loss in a shorter period of time, common to diets with strict induction phases, may predispose you to what I call the "yo-yo phenomenon." While you may lose weight quickly, the odds of putting those pounds back on increase significantly. Shedding pounds rapidly doesn't just make future weight gain more likely however, it also makes subsequent weight loss even more difficult. I can't stress enough that the 10-Step Diet is a *lifestyle* diet, and not some fad diet or a "lose weight quick" scheme. This plan is about your long-term health. Losing weight steadily is an integral part of that equation. When it comes to your total wellness for years to come, there is no rush to the finish line; slow and steady will always win the race. And remember, this could be the last diet book you ever purchase.

Other things to expect as you incorporate each of the steps into your daily routines are a renewed sense of energy, and most likely, a spike in your self-confidence. Being overweight compromises your health, as well as your self-esteem. Whether you have 10 pounds to lose or 100, this diet will help you put the joy and vitality back into your life.

And lastly, expect to reap the rewards of the 10-Step Diet's major benefit. On this diet you will dramatically reduce your chances of chronic disease, including the most devastating—such as heart disease, type 2 diabetes, and cancers. And as this benefit is central to the diet itself, you will find specific dietary and wellness guidelines for ten of the most common and life-threatening diseases Americans face listed in this book.

I want you to lose weight, but more important, I want you to experience the empowering feeling of being in control of your life. From what goes into your mouth to what foods you should avoid in the grocery store, and what you need to know about the connection between disease, weight, and the almost miraculous powers of exercise, there is just no feeling as rewarding as knowing that you are taking steps toward becoming a healthier person, for yourself as well as for the people you love. And since there is no better time than the present, let's begin this journey and make that first step together right now.

Part 1
The 10 Steps

AVOID WHITE CARBS

The Great White Hazards of Dieting and Health

Anyone who has been keeping an eye on the recent nutritional debates knows that almost every diet book talks about carbohydrates—and because of this, there is a tremendous amount of confusion regarding the role carbohydrates should or shouldn't play in nutrition and weight loss. With some diet experts advocating a low-carb diet and others advocating a high-carb diet, how could people *not* be confused?

Scientifically, there's no reason for this debate. The truth is straightforward: not all carbohydrates are created equal. When it comes to weight loss and health, some carbs are good for you (namely, non-starchy vegetables, fruits, whole grains, and beans) and some carbs are bad for you, with none really in between. In light of all this, there is an important distinction to be made between a "low-carb diet" and what I call a *"right-carb diet."*

In the coming pages, my goal is to teach you how to do your carbs right. It is certainly no secret that some foods are better for us than others, but when it comes to carbohydrates and weight loss, this is even more so. It is not just the *quantity* of carbohydrates that matters, but the *quality* as well. A "low-carb diet" restricting nutritious carbs with well-documented health benefits, while still allowing unlimited access to artery-clogging saturated fat, is out of sync with the latest medical science and simply not in the best interest of your health. A "right-carb diet," however, takes full advantage of a bounty of health-promoting vitamins, minerals, phytochemicals, and fiber—and most important, will make your dream of shedding those unwanted pounds into a healthy reality.

You may have guessed that the 10 Step Diet is a right-carb diet. But before we can talk about the right carbs, we have to talk about the *wrong* ones.

White carbohydrates are a dieter's nightmare. Unfortunately, Americans tend to believe that these staples are some of the healthiest food choices available. White potatoes, white rice, white flour, and white flour products (bagels, biscuits, bread, pizza dough, dumplings, pasta, crackers, and countless cereals), along with sugary sweets, have been sabotaging American health for years. (Unfortunately, this list of foods makes up the majority of carbohydrate calories consumed in this country.) As you will see throughout this initial step, the American white carb overload has had grave repercussions on our nation's health. Consumption of these white carbohydrates initiates adverse metabolic changes within our bodies that have been linked to significant weight gain, as well as now-epidemic diseases, including heart disease, type 2 diabetes, and some of the most predominant cancers.

Simply put, white carbs are *not* the "right carbs," and this is why cutting them out of your diet altogether is the very first step you need to take.

The Science Behind Carbohydrates

How your body reacts to various carbohydrate foods isn't rocket science, but it is science—and science you need to understand if you are going to cut these white hazards from your diet once and for all.

The first thing you need to know is that, once broken down in your digestive tract, all carbohydrates (including the right ones) end up in your bloodstream as the same simple molecule—glucose, which is also called blood sugar. The rate at which this process occurs, however, varies drastically depending on the type of carbo-hydrate consumed. Most processed, refined carbs (like the White Hazards) are quickly digested and enter your bloodstream as sugar rapidly. Conversely, most whole food, unrefined carbs, are digested slowly and enter your bloodstream as sugar over a much longer period of time. While the right carbohydrates play a vital role in the body by providing a steady, sustainable energy source chock full of precious vitamins, minerals, and phytochemicals, white carbs—*the wrong carbs*—wreak metabolic havoc because they are so quickly digested. White carbohydrates instigate a cyclical chain of events inside your body that can actually cause you to *gain* weight as opposed to lose it. In fact, because white carbs top the list of quickly digested foods, dieters might as well consider them **public enemy number one.**

So, what is it about white carbs that causes people to gain weight? Well, when you eat white carbs (and other quickly digested carbs), they immediately mainline into your bloodstream as glucose, thus hastily raising your blood sugar. While this may provide you with a quick burst of energy, what happens shortly thereafter can have disastrous effects on your dieting efforts, as well as your health.

This spike in your blood sugar signals your pancreas to release a corresponding surge of insulin. The insulin goes to work doing what it is designed to do: escorting blood sugar from the blood-stream into your cells, where it can be used or stored for energy—

and this is where our dieting efforts begin to get tripped up. To match the blast of sugar that enters the bloodstream after the ingestion of white carbs, your pancreas releases a burst of insulin. As a result of this large and rapid release of insulin, blood glucose is quickly driven from the bloodstream into your cells. The fallout is a precipitous drop in your blood sugar levels. As humans we are genetically hardwired to *despise* low blood sugar, as our brains are completely dependent on glucose for fuel. The brain responds to this precarious situation by awakening its appetite centers. Once roused, those appetite centers order us to go eat; and unfortunately, we tend to eat *more* white carbs, as our bodies know that these are the very foods that will swiftly bring our blood sugar levels back up to an acceptable and comfortable range. In other words, quickly digested white carbs *perpetuate our appetites*. The more we eat them, the more we crave them.

You have probably experienced this sensation after eating a stack of pancakes or some other quickly digested white carbohydrate; two hours after finishing the meal, you start feeling fatigued, lethargic . . . and believe it or not, hungry! If we satisfy these cravings—as most of us will—the whole cycle starts again. Signals from our appetite centers command us to eat foods that spike our blood sugar levels, and the insulin floods our systems once more. We would be better off avoiding this situation altogether.

There is yet another way white carbs, and the blood insulin surges they give rise to, can sabotage your weight loss efforts. Insulin, as the director of fuel management in your body, is a fat-loving, anabolic storage hormone. When it is released into your bloodstream, your fat cells enlarge and store any excess fuel as fat. At the same time, it goes to work opposing the effects of the hormone glucagon, which is responsible for releasing stored fat to be burned for energy. In other words, insulin not only promotes fat storage, but also prevents us from tapping into the fat stores we so badly want to get rid of.

White carbs are *not* the right carbs for weight loss. If you eat a lot of quickly digested carbs and fail to burn the energy they produce, your body will actually fight against your attempts to lose weight and store fat instead.

Understanding the Glycemic Index

Needless to say, if you want to lose weight, there are sound scientific reasons to avoid the *wrong* carbohydrates—those highly refined, quickly digested Great White Hazards. Aside from their white color, how can you tell which carbohydrates are quickly digested and which are slowly digested? Once again, science comes to the rescue with an excellent concept called the glycemic index (GI).

The glycemic index is a measure of how various foods affect your blood sugar level. Foods are ranked on a scale from 0 to 100, according to the extent that they will raise blood sugar levels. Foods that are quickly digested, or rapidly converted into sugar, have a high GI, while foods that are slowly digested have a low glycemic index. Glucose (pure sugar) ranks 100, a baked Russet potato ranks 95, while apples are 38, and lentils 30. Here's a brief list of some common foods and how they rank on the GI.

Baked potato	95
White bread	95
Honey	90
Bagel	72
Watermelon	72
Chocolate bar	70
Corn	70
White rice	70
Bananas	60
Jam	55
Oatmeal	55

Brown rice	50
Peas	50
Carrots	49
Whole grain pasta	40
Strawberries	40
Apples	38
Lentils/dried beans	30
Cherries	22
Soybeans	18
Broccoli	15
Tomatoes	15
Mushrooms	15

It is pretty clear after a good look at this list that the white carbs and the sweetest foods are at the top. On the 10 Step Diet you are only going to eat carbohydrates with a low to moderate GI. In addition, they will all be nutritious and delicious. Your system will digest these foods slowly, thereby ensuring that your energy and blood sugar levels remain steady. Furthermore, foods with a lower GI ranking will not flood your system with insulin, so the cycle of blood sugar peaks and valleys will not be activated.

It is impractical and unnecessary to feel compelled to memorize the GI of each and every food you eat. Simply remember that the White Hazards all have a high glycemic index and that most beans, whole grains, non-starchy vegetables, and non-tropical fruits (all "right" carbs) have a low to moderate glycemic index.

Beware of Insulin Resistance—How Fat Begets More Fat

One of the unhealthiest consequences of having excess body fat, or gaining weight in general, is how it affects the action of insulin, the body's fuel-storage hormone. When we gain weight, especially in our abdominal areas, complex biochemical changes take place that alter how our cells respond to insulin. Specifically, our cells become less responsive, or *resistant*, to insulin's effects. This situation is aptly called insulin resistance syndrome.

In order to understand the ramifications of insulin resistance, think of insulin as a key and its receptor as a lock. If you change the shape of the lock (receptor), the key (insulin) will no longer fit. If insulin does not fit into its receptor correctly, the fuel it normally delivers to your cells, namely blood sugar and blood fats, cannot enter. Thus, blood sugar and blood fat levels continue to rise, in turn, prompting the pancreas to unleash even more insulin into the bloodstream. In other words, the pancreas attempts to compensate for insulin's inability to perform its function by secreting more insulin than it normally would. This creates a relative state of insulin excess in the bloodstream known as hyperinsulinemia, the biochemical marker for insulin resistance syndrome. Knowing that insulin is a fat-storing hormone, it should come as no surprise that hyperinsulinemia is associated with obesity, and if you have this condition, white carbs only add potent fuel to insulin's fat-storing fire. In addition to promoting stubborn obesity, insulin resistance syndrome dramatically increases your risk of type 2 diabetes and all forms of cardiovascular disease.

Unfortunately, until you manage to get it under control, this condition will mitigate your weight loss efforts; however, the good news is that there are several simple and effective interventions you can employ to break free of insulin resistance forever. As we go through the 10 Steps of this diet, you will learn about each of these important, life-saving strategies, but at the moment, know that the most important specific dietary strategy to overcome insulin resistance is to categorically avoid white carbs. For most people with insulin resistance, avoiding white carbs, along with a few other dietary and lifestyle changes, clears up the abnormal biochemistry precipitating the condition.

It is important for your weight loss endeavors, as well as your health in general, to determine whether or not you have this metabolic condition. Your healthcare provider can order a blood insulin level; however, it can frequently be identified by referring to the markers for insulin resistance listed here.

- High blood triglycerides
- Low HDL (good) cholesterol
- A fat belly (waist size greater than 35 inches in women and 40 inches in men) or a tendency to gain weight in the mid section
- Having type 2 diabetes or a positive family history
- Elevated blood pressure
- Elevated LDL cholesterol
- Difficulty losing weight
- A history of coronary artery disease

If you have even one of these markers, your chances of having insulin resistance are significant. If you have two or more markers, the likelihood of having some degree of insulin resistance is very high. **Remember, in this instance, it is critical that you avoid white carbs at all costs.**

Tricks of the Trade

Of course, sometimes life happens. It would be unreasonable not to assume that eventually you will find yourself in a situation where you'll *have* to eat—or *want* to eat—a high glycemic index carb. When this happens, the best course of action is to counter the harmful blood sugar/insulin response by eating strategically. If you have to eat a high GI carb, pair it with another food that will slow its digestion. Remember, when you slow digestion you naturally slow down how quickly that carb will enter your bloodstream as glucose. When you indulge in a high GI carb this simple strategy can spare you some of the consequences of blood glucose and insulin surges.

Protein, fiber, fat, and acidic foods, such as lemon or vinegar, can all effectively prolong the digestive process. A practical application of this helpful bit of nutritional science is to combine your popcorn snack with a stick of string cheese (protein). Or, if you want toast for breakfast, use a little almond butter (good fat) as a spread. Can't avoid having a baked potato? Then make sure to eat it along with a mixed meal: chicken breast (protein) and tossed salad (fiber) with olive oil (good fat) and vinegar (acid) dressing. Eat the potato skin, too, for that much more fiber.

Two Notable White Carb Exceptions

If the thought of banishing all white carbs and starches doesn't sit right with you, I have good news. You can indulge in special forms of white bread and white rice that will not send your blood sugar and insulin levels surging upward. Authentic sourdough bread, because it is acidic, and Uncle Ben's converted white rice, because of its starch structure, actually rank relatively low on the glycemic index. Sourdough bread has a GI of 52, compared to the GI of 95 for French baguette; Uncle Ben's converted white rice has a GI of 44, compared to a GI of 72 for short grain white rice.

Although these unique white carbs have a more favorable GI, they do provide slightly more calories per serving, along with fewer minerals and less fiber than true whole grains (see Step 2); eat these allowable white carbs in moderation for that occasional white carb fix.

Health Matters

There is another big reason to avoid the Great White Hazards—your good health depends on it. Too much insulin pumping through your bloodstream not only sabotages your weight loss, but it can also have devastating effects upon your health. Thanks to scientific studies we now know about an ominous connection between high glycemic white carbohydrates and heart disease, type 2 diabetes, and even some cancers.

Heart Disease

Over the past decade, medical studies have confirmed that having an elevated blood insulin level (hyperinsulinemia) is strongly associated with increased cardiovascular risk. In fact, among heart attack victims, insulin resistance—and the high blood insulin levels accompanying it—is a more common feature than smoking, high blood pressure, or even high cholesterol.

How could it be that insulin, the hormone that plays such a fundamental and vital role in furnishing our cells with energy, betrays us so when secreted into the bloodstream in excess? The complete answer involves a great deal of complicated and complex biochemistry—some of which you read above—but there is a simple summary available, too. It is what I call the "insulin quadruple heart whammy." Having too much insulin in the bloodstream as a result of over consuming refined white carbs is associated with the following four aspects of heart disease:

1. An elevation in blood pressure
2. An elevation in triglycerides (a dangerous blood fat)
3. A lowering of the protective, HDL (good) cholesterol
4. A dysfunction of the cells lining our arteries.

Take heart and stay away from those refined, high glycemic, white carbohydrates that will adeptly permeate your arteries with too much insulin.

Type 2 Diabetes

Risk factors for the development of this epidemic, potentially life-threatening condition include being overweight, being physically inactive, having a close relative with the disease, and consuming trans fats. If you have any of these traits, it is imperative that you avoid regular consumption of the Great White Hazards. Results from the highly esteemed, Harvard University based Nurses' Health

Study confirm these are the foods eaten most commonly by people who develop type 2 diabetes (*Journal of the American Medical Association*, February 12, 1997, Volume 227 (6)).

The underlying metabolic problem in type 2 diabetes is insulin resistance. Victims of type 2 diabetes typically suffer from some degree of insulin resistance for many years prior to developing the disease in full. If your insulin doesn't work well and you eat high glycemic white carbs, your pancreas is forced to release that much more insulin to get all of the blood sugar into your cells.

Repeating this scenario over time eventually outstrips the supply of insulin the pancreas is capable of producing. As a result, you have inadequate blood insulin levels, and your cells are not able to take up the blood glucose they need to survive. When your blood glucose rises too high, you have developed full-blown type 2 diabetes.

Cancer

The *sine qua non* of all cancer is uncontrolled cellular growth. Any factor that promotes cellular growth in the body can increase the likelihood that a cell will become cancerous. Consuming the wrong carbs may just be such a factor. In fact, many studies have shown a positive association between the "typical western diet" and some of the most life-threatening cancers. One of the defining features of a westernized diet is that it is high in refined, high glycemic carbohydrates. Although the exact relationship between eating lots of refined carbs and increasing your cancer risk has not been fully elucidated, many scientists speculate the answer lies with the infamous blood insulin level. Cells in the body proliferate more readily when stimulated by hormones called insulin-like-growth-factors (IGFs).

Laboratory studies have specifically shown that cells of the prostate, colon, and breast respond to insulin-like-growth-factor-1 (IGF-1). As the name suggests, the trigger for the release of IGF-1 is insulin itself. Hyperinsulinemia may lead to excessive IGF-1 production. Too much IGF-1 may lead to excessive cellular proliferation in these tissues, and ultimately, to cancer itself. A recent study published in the *Journal of the National Cancer Institute* (February 4, 2004, Volume 96 (3)) reported that women who consumed the highest glycemic diets were nearly three times more likely to develop colon cancer, compared to women with the lowest glycemic diets.

Another scientific finding suggesting that elevated blood insulin promotes cancer comes from a provocative study published in the *New England Journal of Medicine* (April 24, 2003, Volume 348 (17)). This study found that being overweight may account for 20 percent of cancer deaths in women and 14 percent of cancer deaths in men. That is a sum total of 900,000 cancer deaths, due to being overweight, in this country annually. Investigators hypothesize that an elevated blood insulin level, common in those with excess body fat, may very well be one of the reasons for their observations.

No matter how much you love your white carbs, you need to make every effort to rid them from your diet. Losing weight without losing the white carbs is virtually impossible; but if that is not catalyst enough, consider the many health risks associated with overconsumption of high glycemic carbohydrates. Believe it or not, once you cut these foods from your diet, you will barely miss them. Instead of craving the *wrong* carbs, such as a baked potato or a hunk of white bread, you will begin to crave the *right* carbs, including beans, whole grains, non-starchy vegetables, and fruits. And trust me—the ease with which you will start to lose weight, along with the health benefits you are sure to reap, will be worth all the effort this initial step might take.

Step 1 Action Plan: Avoid the Great White Hazard

Strictly avoid:

1. White flour and products containing it, such as: white bread, biscuits, rolls, bagels, pretzels, dumplings, pancakes, waffles, pizza, many cereals, and crackers.
2. White potatoes whether mashed, boiled, or baked. Also avoid French fries and potato chips.
3. White rice and other rice products, such as rice cakes and puffed rice cereals.
4. Sugar/sweets: cookies, cakes, pastries, donuts, candy, pies, ice cream, and sodas.

Make sure to read the labels! White flour is generally referred to as "wheat flour" or "enriched wheat flour" on food labels.

EAT THE RIGHT CARBS:
MIRACLE BEANS AND GREAT GRAINS

Enjoying the Right Carbs

As you know by now, I am not an advocate of a "no-carb" or "low-carb diet," but rather, a big believer in a *"right-carb diet."* When it comes to maximizing your state of wellness and increasing the probability of permanent and successful weight loss, learning how to do your carbs right is one of the most powerful nutritional strategies you can incorporate into your daily life.

Now that we have tackled the *wrong* carbs, we can start discussing the four delicious categories of *right* carbs: non-starchy vegetables, fruits, whole grains, and beans. These carbohydrates contain a bounty of health-promoting vitamins, minerals, fiber, and disease-fighting phytochemicals. Plus, unlike the Great White Hazards, they are digested slowly, resulting in a more prolonged and gentle glucose/insulin response.

We will discuss fruits and vegetables at length in Step 5, but at the moment, I want to introduce you to the other right carbs: miracle beans and great grains. By consuming an abundance of non-starchy vegetables and beans, modest amounts of whole grains and fruit, and minimal to no refined white carbs, you will lower your risk of heart disease, improve your gastrointestinal health, lower your risk of a host of cancers, protect against type 2 diabetes, and lose weight!

Miracle Beans

With over twenty-four varieties available, beans are perhaps the most underutilized "diet food" there is. Beans, along with peas and lentils, are members of the legume family of vegetables. They are not only remarkably good for you, but also incredibly versatile and economical. No matter which variety you prefer, beans are rich in healthy vegetable protein and fiber and low in fat. The only exception to this rule is the peanut and soybean, which have similar amounts of protein and fiber, but fewer carbohydrates and a generous quantity of "healthy fat."

Overall, beans are an outstanding source of micronutrients. They provide several important minerals, including a generous supply of iron, magnesium, and potassium. Beans are an excellent source of the B vitamins, such as riboflavin, thiamine, niacin, and folate. In fact, beans can proudly boast being one of the richest dietary sources of folate—now famous for its heart-healthy and cancer-protective attributes.

Like fruits and vegetables, beans are also loaded with phytochemicals, including flavonoids, one of the most powerful classes of antioxidant and disease-fighting phytochemicals. *The Journal of Agricultural and Food Chemistry* (December 31, 2003) reports that of twelve varieties of beans, black beans offer the greatest amount of flavonoids, followed by red, brown, yellow, and white beans. Interestingly, this data is perfectly consistent with what we already know to be true about the antioxidant power of fruits and vegetables—the more colorful the food, the more powerful it is.

With their unique combination of high protein and high fiber (higher than any other category of "right carb"), beans offer slower digestion and a gradual, more sustained blood glucose response. Collectively, beans have the second lowest glycemic index of the four categories of *right* carbs; non-starchy vegetables have the lowest glycemic index, and fruits and whole grains tie for third place. Besides nutritiously satisfying your appetite, beans can also lower your cholesterol, protect your heart, and help stabilize your blood insulin level if you are insulin resistant.

There are some great and easy ways to incorporate beans into your diet. Replace the *wrong* carbs with the *right* ones, and try a side of beans instead of white carbs, such as pasta, potatoes, or rice. Another great bean trick is to puree them, making a tasty dip or sandwich spread. If you need an even easier way to get beans into your diet, just toss them into your salad. Canned beans are super-convenient, but generally contain lots of sodium. Always drain and rinse them with water to remove as much sodium as possible. Most people agree that dried beans, when freshly prepared, have a superior texture and flavor; and keep in mind that most dried beans can be prepared in a pressure cooker in about twenty minutes. Having a pressure cooker on hand is a simple way to dramatically increase the frequency of your bean consumption. Lentils, some of the healthiest legumes, cook far more quickly than dried beans, and can be prepared on the stove top in fifteen to twenty minutes.

The Side Effect of Beans

Some people suffer from gas when they eat beans. When your digestive enzymes are unable to break down all of the starch contained in beans, the bacteria in your colon will often ferment the remnants. Gas is a natural by-product of this fermentation process. If you are one of the unfortunate individuals who experiences this uncomfortable (and occasionally embarrassing) situation, try these gas-troubleshooting tips:

· Consume the beans/legumes known to cause the least amount of gas—lima beans, Anasazi, black eyed peas, chick peas, mung beans, split peas, and lentils.

· Discard the cooking liquid and rinse beans in fresh water before consuming them.

· Rinse canned beans thoroughly.

· Don't consume a large quantity of beans in one sitting.

· Use a pressure cooker.

· Consider using Beano or another over-the-counter digestive enzyme product.

Great Grains

The next category of healthy, permissible carbs is whole grains. At one time or another, even some of the Great White Hazards were "Great Grains." When grains are refined and processed to produce products like white flour or white rice, the outer coat or bran and inner germ portions are removed; this process effectively strips the grains of their fiber and their innate nutritional value. Consequently, it is much easier for your digestive system to rapidly turn them into glucose. Because whole grains do not go through this refinement process, they remain intact and retain their outer bran coat (a rich source of fiber and minerals) and their inner germ (a dense package of vitamin E, B vitamins, and phytochemicals). The good news is that your digestive system has to work longer and harder to process whole grains. The sugar, which they eventually break down to, will not rush into our bloodstreams, as it does when we consume refined grains such as white flour and white rice.

A recent Harvard study found that among 74,000 women, those who consumed the most fiber-rich grains, such as oatmeal and whole-grain cereals, gained less weight over time than women who consumed the least amount of fiber in their diets (*American Journal of Clinical Nutrition*, November 2003, Volume 78 (5)). A second Harvard based study with 86,000 males over the age of forty found that the more whole grain cereals a man consumed, the less likely he was to die from cardiovascular disease or any other cause (*American Journal of Clinical Nutrition*, March 2003; Volume 77 (3)).

There are many different varieties of whole grains to choose from. Yet, even though whole wheat, whole oats, rye, barley, buckwheat, quinoa, and brown rice are brimming with health-promoting nutrients and generous amounts of fiber, we can't forget about the glycemic index. Like most fruits, these great grains have a *moderate* glycemic index ranking—not a *low* glycemic index ranking. For this reason, I suggest you pair your grain products (bread, cereals, snacks) with another food that provides additional fiber, healthy fat, protein, or acid. Remember, these are the four food components that can slow digestion or lower the glycemic index of a carbohydrate food. I suggest having your whole grain cereal topped with wheat germ (extra fiber) or freshly ground flax (extra fiber/fat) and skim or soy milk (protein). Enjoy whole grain tortilla chips dipped in hummus (protein, fiber). Dip a slice of freshly baked whole grain bread in extra virgin olive oil (healthy fat).

It is also worth noting that some grains have a lower GI than others. Although the reasons are not totally understood, studies have shown that all types of rye bread, regardless of the amount of fiber they contain, produce a lower insulin response than wheat bread. Whole grain rye bread is a great choice.

Of course, knowing what you are eating is sometimes a difficult task; when it comes to great grains, you want to make sure that the products you select are truly "whole grains." Currently, food labeling laws in the U.S. are such that any grain product containing 51 percent intact grains can be deemed "whole grain." If you want to be assured you are getting only "whole grain," and not a refined counterpart (such as white flour), make sure the label says "100 percent whole grain." If you see "wheat flour," "enriched wheat flour," or any other grain without "whole" written in front of it, it's nothing more than refined flour disguised as the healthier option!

It is vital to your health and weight loss endeavors to swap out the wrong carbs for the right ones. By eating beans and whole grains in lieu of those high glycemic carbs we discussed in Step 1, you will be taking proactive steps to meeting your own weight loss goals and protecting your health.

Step 2 Action Plan: Eat the Right Carbs

Miracle Beans Plan of Action

1. Strive to have one serving of beans a day.
2. Although all beans/legumes (with the exception of fava beans, which have a very high GI) are permissible on the 10 Step Diet, concentrate your efforts on the lowest glycemic index dieting superstars—soybeans, lentils, kidney beans, chickpeas (garbanzo beans), butter beans, navy beans, black beans, white beans, and split peas.

Great Grains Plan of Action

1. When consuming grain products (bread, cereals, crackers, etc.) make sure they are **100 percent whole grain.** Please note, you *must* see "whole" before "grain" (for example, whole wheat, whole oat, whole barley) on the ingredients label; otherwise the grain is refined.
2. Always have your grain products with foods containing either protein, healthy fat, fiber, or acid to further reduce their glycemic index.
3. Concentrate on the lowest glycemic index dieting superstars: oats, barley, rye/pumpernickel.

DUMP THE LIQUID CALORIES

Are Liquid Calories Drowning Your Diet?

Of all the things you can do to improve your health and meet your weight loss goals, this simple step might offer the single greatest return for your efforts. Liquid calories can make or break your attempts to lose weight. In fact, liquid calories may actually be more fattening or cause weight gain more readily than their solid food counterparts. Whether you are partial to sports drinks, sodas, or fruit drinks, each time you quench your thirst with one of these popular beverages, you are consuming calories derived almost entirely from sugar. At this point, you know that sugary beverages have a high glycemic index. In fact, liquid sugars bypass the digestive process altogether, zipping straight into your bloodstream.

The average 12-ounce soda contains about 150 calories, offers absolutely no nutritional value, and because it is liquid, provides minimal volume effect in your stomach. As we will discuss later, physical bulk within the gastrointestinal tract, something you do not get with liquid calories, plays an important role in appetite suppression. But that's not the worst of it. Essentially all of the calories in soda (and most sweetened beverages) are derived from a particularly sinister invention of modern food technology called high fructose corn syrup (HFCS). Developed in the early seventies, this versatile liquid sweetener is 75 percent sweeter and less expensive than sugar; as such, it has significantly contributed to the staggering increase in the availability and consumption of sweetened, processed foods and beverages in this country. Recent studies show that our biological systems don't respond to HFCS in an orthodox fashion; as a result, HFCS may be more readily converted to fat. According to Dr. George Bray, an eminent and highly respected obesity scientist at Louisiana State University, "It is a carbohydrate fat equivalent." A study published in the April 2004 issue of the *American Journal of Clinical Nutrition* (Volume 79 (4)), reveals a strong association between the increased use of HFCS in the seventies and eighties and the development of the American obesity epidemic.

Consider this: if you drink one 12-ounce soda daily (that's 150 calories), over and above the calories you expend, you will gain 15 pounds in one year. Stated another way, if you stop drinking that 12-ounce can of soda and otherwise maintain your current level of caloric consumption, you can lose 15 pounds in one year. Most popular carbonated beverages contain the equivalent of 9 teaspoons of sugar per serving. Would you ever put 9 teaspoons of sugar in your coffee or cereal?

Alas, because your complete health is at the core of the 10-Step Diet, I must tell you that diet sodas are an unacceptable replacement. All carbonated beverages, even diet brands, are acidic in nature. The acids from carbonated beverages enter your bloodstream and need to be buffered. In these instances, calcium comes to the rescue—but to neutralize these acids, the calcium frequently has to exit your bones. When bones lose calcium they become weaker. Teeth fare even worse than bones. A recent British study among 1,753 twelve-year-olds found that even having one serving of carbonated beverages a day significantly increases tooth enamel erosion; drinking four or more servings a day raises the chances of tooth enamel erosion by 252 percent (*British Dental Journal*, March 13, 2004, Volume 196 (5)).

Believe it or not, these so-called diet drinks may actually result in weight gain, despite their zero calorie make up. It seems that for some of us, the mere taste of something sweet in our mouths can trigger a blood/insulin response. If you are one of these unlucky individuals and you nurse two or three diet sodas throughout the day, you may be repeatedly priming your bloodstream with insulin, that wily fat-storage hormone. One of my clients lost 12 pounds in two months simply by giving up his daily diet colas. If you are hooked on diet sodas, work on weaning yourself off of them; they are simply not healthy beverages.

The Info on H2O

There is one, and only one, beverage that is perfectly suited to our biological needs—pure, clean, natural water. I have seen countless patients successfully lose weight just by substituting water for sodas and other sugar-fortified beverages. Water is your body's most vital essential nutrient, and it is especially good for those who need and want to lose weight.

It seems logical that regular water consumption helps us feel fuller, but until recently there was little conclusive evidence that drinking lots of water would definitely hasten weight loss. A new study, conducted among six men and six women by German researchers, shows that drinking water *does* increase the rate at which people burn calories. According to their findings, published in *The Journal of Clinical Endocrinology and Metabolism* (December 2003, Volume 88 (12)), after drinking 17 ounces of water, the subjects' metabolic rates—the rate at which calories are burned—transiently increased by 30 percent. The researchers estimate that over a one year period of time, a person who increases his water intake by 1.5 liters a day would burn an extra 17,400 calories, which is equivalent to a weight loss of 5 pounds.

Make sure the water you drink is pure and clean. If you have any questions about the safety and quality of your municipal water supply, drink bottled water or consider purchasing a home water purification system. When it comes to your health, this is a small investment.

Toasting to Good Health

Is alcohol allowed on the 10-Step Diet? Certainly, as long as it's the right kind and the right amount. Many studies have now confirmed that alcohol in moderation can significantly diminish the risk of heart attacks and ischemic strokes. Although all forms of alcohol have been shown to benefit our hearts and arteries, for weight loss, some are better than others. A glass of wine, 1.5 ounces of spirits, or a low-carb/light beer is permissible. Stay away from all regular beer. Maltose, the carbohydrate in beer, can raise your blood sugar level faster than any other food, except a baked potato. The classic "beer belly" is an accurate visual depiction of what overconsumption of high glycemic foods and beverages does to our bodies.

For those who enjoy alcohol, but still want to lose weight, there is good news from Harvard's Nurses' Health Study II (*Diabetes Care*, July 2003, Volume 26 (7)). Researchers found that moderate alcohol consumption in overweight women actually has a positive impact on blood sugar and insulin levels. Meaning, it appears to improve insulin's sensitivity. That's healthy, important news for those who are unwilling to part with their daily glass of wine and suffer from insulin resistance.

Red wine has special features that deserve mention. It is loaded with a potent class of antioxidant phytochemicals called phenolics. Promising data from laboratory studies have shown these substances might reduce heart disease and cancer. The darkest and most astringent red wines are the true antioxidant stars: most merlots, cabernet sauvignons, red zinfandels, and syrahs/shirazes.

Although the 10-Step Diet permits up to one *right* alcoholic beverage a day, all forms of alcohol contain calories that you probably don't need. It is foolish to feel compelled to start drinking for your health, when you will likely reach your weight loss goals more quickly if you avoid these liquid calories entirely.

A Spot of Tea

For cultures around the world and centuries over, tea has been *the* primary beverage of choice. But this popular beverage doesn't just have staying power; it also has proven health benefits. Dr. John Weisburger, a researcher at the American Health Foundation, believes tea is one of the easiest and quickest ways to infuse our bodies and brains with antioxidants. It is so beneficial that Dr. Weisburger believes "tea should be the national health beverage."

Tea is especially rich in a potent class of antioxidants called polyphenols. Of these polyphenols, EGCG proves to be one of the most impressive antioxidants ever documented. In fact, brewed tea appears to have more antioxidant power than almost any vegetable or fruit. Laboratory and epidemiologic studies show that regular tea consumption may protect the cardiovascular system, the immune system, and offer general protection from cancers.

This message was brought home in a 2003 report to the Proceedings of the National Academy of Sciences (May 13, 2003, volume 100 (10)): non-tea drinkers who drank five to six cups of black tea per day for two weeks appeared better equipped to fight off bacterial infection than those who did not drink black tea at all. Apparently, there is an ingredient common to black, green, oolong, and pekoe teas that boosts the immune system's ability to attack harmful bacteria. Of course, this doesn't mean tea-drinkers will never get sick, but it does mean that they may have a milder case of infection if they do.

To get the most benefit from tea it is best to brew your own—particularly black or green tea, both of which contain the most antioxidants. Always steep for at least two minutes and gently squeeze the loose tea to "wring out" as many antioxidants as possible. Unfortunately, research has shown that herbal teas, powdered tea mixes, and commercial bottled teas do not contain significant amounts of antioxidants. Decaffeinated loose teas provide some antioxidants, but not as much as the regular variety.

Getting Juiced from Juices

What about fruit juices? While 100 percent fruit juices can certainly offer a concentrated source of vitamins and minerals, unfortunately, they also provide a concentrated source of sugar and calories. One cup of orange juice typically contains the sugar from three or more oranges, and as you know now, sugar in liquid form will zoom right into your bloodstream without hesitation. Alas, this spike in your blood sugar will set you up for hunger later. Remember, the glycemic index of fruit juice is *always* higher than whole fruits, where the sugars are bound up in all the fiber a piece of fruit offers. Instead, try a glass of tomato juice or V8.

Step 3 Action Plan: Dump the Liquid Calories

1. Drink pure, clean water as your primary beverage. Have a goal of drinking six or more 8-ounce glasses a day.
2. Avoid sodas, fruit juices, fruit drinks, sports drinks, chocolate milk, sugar-sweetened tea, and any other sweet tasting liquids.

Enjoy these permissible beverages:
1. 100% vegetable juice—tomato/V8
2. Coffee
3. Organic soy milk
4. Unsweetened tea
5. 1% or skim milk
6. Wine (red is best), 5 ounces or less a day
7. Low-carb or light beer, 12 ounces or less a day
8. Spirits, 1.5 ounces a day or less, straight or with a non-caloric mixer (soda/water)

STEP 4

CONTROL YOUR PORTIONS

The Truth About Portion Distortion

It seems as though weight loss in America grows more complex with every passing year. Currently, 64 percent of the American population is overweight, with 30 percent considered clinically obese. If we compare the advertising budget of McDonald's to that of the U.S. Government, there is no denying that the good guys are outnumbered and outspent. McDonald's spends one billion dollars a year hoping to convince us to stop at their drive-through windows on our way home from work, while the U.S. Government has a meager thirty million dollars a year to promote healthy eating habits.

The truth is Americans are pressured to overeat—and because of this pressure, we are eating more than ever before. According to the USDA, we consume 140 to 200 more calories a day than we did twenty years ago. Assuming that our activity levels have remained the same, this increase in caloric intake translates into an additional

14 to 20 pounds of weight gain annually for every man, woman, and child in this country. "Portion distortion" is a major reason we are now one of the heaviest nations in the world.

According to a report in the *Journal of the American Medical Association* (January 22, 2003, Volume 289 (4)), between 1977 and 1998 portion sizes increased for all foods served at home and in restaurants with the exception of pizza. Within our overwhelming, bigger-is-better (and frequently cheaper) food culture, we must make a constant, conscious effort to control our portions; and we need to be vigilant about it.

Portion control is fundamental to dieting and weight maintenance and absolutely paramount to good health in general. While every step of the 10-Step Diet will play an important role in maximizing your wellness and achieving your weight loss goal, this step needs to transcend all aspects of your food-related behavior.

Before you read any further, I want you to put this book down and cup your two hands together. Believe it or not, this is the approximate size and capacity of your stomach. Whenever you are in doubt about the amount of food you should eat, perform this simple exercise. It is a very useful visual guide to help you keep your portions on target.

Whether you are buying food, ordering food, preparing food, or serving food—think *portion control*. With the exception of non-starchy vegetables—which you can supersize at will—I recommend that you never consume more than the capacity of your cupped hands at any one sitting. That said, don't start worrying that you will be hungry all the time; as mentioned in the introduction, the 10 Step Diet is designed to keep your hunger at bay. Remember that part of the problem dieters face is that hunger can override willpower. If you faithfully follow all 10 Steps, I guarantee you will always feel pleasantly satisfied, which will make the all-important step of controlling your portions easier than you could ever imagine.

Unfortunately, when it comes to diet books, Americans are frequently misled. Yes, as many report, the specific *kind of food* we eat is important for losing weight, but so is the *amount of food* we eat. It is a shame that so many "health gurus" feel compelled to distort this truth. If there is one hard and fast rule to weight loss, it is—and will always be—you must eat fewer calories than you burn. For most of us, this means adjusting the portion sizes to which we have become accustomed. If you want to achieve permanent and successful weight loss, you simply must control the amount of food that goes on your plate and into your body. This is especially important in current times. The American Institute of Cancer Research (July 17, 2003) reports that Americans can, and do, unconsciously take in more calories—as much as 56 percent more—when served bigger portions.

According to the National Institute of Health, here's how our current "portion distortion" stacks up against what we ate twenty years ago:

- On average, a bagel was 3 inches in diameter and had 140 calories. Today, a typical bagel is 6 inches across and has a hefty 350 calories.
- The customary cheeseburger had 333 calories. Today, your favorite eat will cost you 590 calories. (This means you'll have to lift weights one and a half hours to burn up those extra 257 calories.)
- The traditional cup of spaghetti with sauce and three meatballs was 500 calories. Sit down today at any Italian eatery and you'll likely dive into a whopping 1,025 calories.
- In previous years, an ordinary serving of french fries was about 2.4 ounces, and it had about 210 calories. Bad news: the standard helpings are now 6.9 ounces and have 610 calories.
- Twenty years ago, the usual turkey sandwich had 320 calories. Today, you'll gobble up as many as 820 calories.

Perhaps the most frightening aspect of all this is that we humans are notorious for eating everything placed before us. A 2001 study conducted at Penn State University served lunch to study participants on four separate occasions. Over the course of the experiment, the main dish increased in size—from 500 to 625 grams, 625 to 750 grams, and finally, from 750 to 1,000 grams. Despite having the same level of hunger prior to each lunchtime meal, the participants consistently ate more as the portion sizes increased (*Science Now*, Winter 2004, Volume 7).

But if a portion is what will fit into your two hands when cupped together, then what is a *serving*? Like portion distortion, Americans have completely lost sight of normal serving sizes. Awareness and ultilization of appropriate serving sizes is an **essential component** of establishing and maintaining optimal weight. Think back to Step 2: Eating the Right Carbs. Remember that you should have a serving of beans daily—that's a half cup. For Great Grains a serving is one slice of bread or a half cup of brown rice. Here is a list of guidelines for other food groups as well.

- A basic fruit, non-leafy vegetable, grain, or bean serving size is a half cup, or about the size of your fist.
- A serving of animal protein is 3 ounces—the size of a deck of playing cards.
- Whole grain bread—one slice.
- Dairy products—6 ounces of yogurt, 1 cup of milk, and 1 ounce of cheese, which is the size of your thumb.
- Oil—only what fits in 1 tablespoon.

Step 4 Action Plan: Portion Control

1. Remember that the capacity of your stomach is equivalent to your two hands cupped together. Don't consume more than this at any one sitting. (Non-starchy vegetables are an exception.)

2. Keep in mind that we are bad judges of whether or not we are full. To circumvent this genetic shortcoming, don't put too much food on your plate, and eat slowly.

3. When dining out, remember, virtually all eating establishments with the general exception of those featuring healthy or fine cuisine, serve enough for two or more people. Take a proactive approach and request smaller portions. Don't be afraid of asking the waitstaff to package half of your meal in a carry-away box before they serve it to you—think of it this way, it's two meals for the price of one!

4. See Step 10 for snacking strategies. "Controlled grazing" will help keep your hunger at bay and decrease your desire to overeat.

LOAD UP ON VEGGIES
(AND HAVE A LITTLE FRUIT, TOO)

Nature's Megastars

If the empty calories of sugar-fortified drinks are a dieter's night-mare, then this potent food group is a dieter's dream. Of course, in this day and age, everyone knows that fruits and vegetables are good for us—but in this step, I want to make sure you know just how good they are and why. As I have said throughout the 10 Step Diet, the people who have the greatest weight loss successes are those who understand why they should eat certain foods and avoid others. If you happen to be someone who doesn't take advantage of the extraordinary health and weight loss benefits of fruits and veggies, I hope this step will change your life for the better.

Veggies

Let's start with vegetables—the ideal food for a dieter. You have probably already surmised the first reason: non-starchy vegetables have a very low glycemic index. As you know by now, this means non-starchy vegetables, even when eaten in large quantities, are not going to activate the blood insulin surges that increase your appetite and throw your body into fat-storage mode. Furthermore, veggies are the quintessential "big food"; they supply lots of bulk from fiber and water and very little in the form of calories. This is an important point; outside of calories, the only other thing that can suppress a human's appetite is volume or actual physical bulk from food in the stomach. In this regard, vegetables rule. You can fill up on a platter piled high with broccoli and still consume no more than 100 calories in the process. As a health conscious dieter, vegetables give you the most bang for your buck, and due to their low-caloric makeup there is no such thing as Step 4 portion control with vegetables. When eaten in abundance, these super healthy, super bulky, low-cal foods help maintain a steady blood glucose level, keep your stomach feeling full, and ultimately, keep your brain's appetite centers quiet.

On the 10-Step Diet you can eat as many non-starchy vegetables as you desire—pile them on your dinner plate, eat a big healthy salad for lunch, put some onions and peppers in your eggs in the morning—you name it. Remember, too, that vegetables are the perfect between-meal snack. Try some carrots dipped in hummus or celery sticks spread with peanut butter.

But these are just the reasons vegetables make good diet foods—I have yet to say anything about the health-promoting benefits they offer.

Recent health and nutrition studies are showing that vegetables are better for us than we ever imagined. For over a half century we have known that vegetables are bursting with health promoting fiber, vitamins, and minerals, but in the last twenty years we have discovered that they are also loaded with an extraordinary group of disease busting agents called phytochemicals. Plants produce these substances to protect themselves against a host of environmental threats—from damaging ultraviolet radiation to plant-eating parasites. Fortunately, it turns out that these same plant-protective substances are just as good for humans. Several thousand phytochemicals have been identified thus far, and they perform truly spectacular feats in our bodies with the greatest of ease. In fact, the pharmaceutical industry can only dream of producing drugs capable of performing as effectively in our systems as phytochemicals do. What's even more exciting is that scientists estimate that there are up to one hundred thousand of these chemicals still to be characterized.

Phytochemicals protect our bodies against disease in a myriad of ways, but they are most valuable for their antioxidant, detoxifying, anti-inflammatory, and immune boosting powers. If you think that you are getting these life-preserving chemicals from a supplement or a sports bar—in lieu of vegetables—then be forewarned. These miraculous agents of good health are only found in plant-based foods, namely fruits, vegetables, whole grains, beans, nuts, and seeds. Thus, a diet chock-full of vegetables will not only help you lose weight, but also help you ward off heart attacks, strokes, high blood pressure, gastrointestinal diseases, cataracts, macular degeneration, as well as a host of cancers. Moreover, because fruits and vegetables boast the highest concentration of phytochemicals, they are the ideal food group for a leaner look and better health overall. So much so, that it is worth taking a closer look at what some of these phytochemicals do for our bodies.

> **The Superstar Veggies for Wellness and Weight Loss**
>
> · All of the cruciferous class—broccoli, cabbage, kale, collards, cauliflower, brussels sprouts, and watercress
>
> · Carrots
>
> · Garlic
>
> · Onions and leeks
>
> · Tomatoes
>
> · Bell peppers—red, yellow, orange
>
> · Asparagus
>
> · Spinach and darker lettuces

The Power of Feisty Phytochemicals

Although you may not have recognized them as phytochemicals, many of you are likely familiar with some of the commonly known superstars such as lycopene in tomatoes, anthocyanins in berries, and sulforaphane in broccoli. I am certain that a brief profile of just these three amazing plant chemicals will motivate you to eat your vegetables with robust enthusiasm.

Lycopene is the phytochemical pigment in **tomatoes** that gives them their vivid red color and is one of the most potent antioxidants known. Antioxidants are scavengers of rogue molecules called *free radicals*, which run around in our bodies initiating a cascade of damaging oxidation. Free radicals are by-products of the body's normal metabolic processes, although they can also enter our bodies from environmental sources like tobacco smoke, chemicals, smog, prescription drugs, ultraviolet radiation, and even the foods we eat. Unfortunately, the oxidation induced by free radicals damages vital cellular structures and ultimately contributes to the development of cancer, heart disease, cataracts, arthritis, skin wrinkling, and even the aging process itself. Because cancer can result from a deficiency of antioxidants, and lycopene is such a powerful antioxidant, it is not surprising that studies from around the word have revealed general cancer protection from diets rich in tomatoes.

As an anticancer agent, Lycopene seems to protect the prostate the most zealously, which is interesting to note as this phytochemical seems to concentrate in this particular part of the body. A Harvard based study published in the *Journal of the National Cancer Institute* (December 6, 1995, Volume 87 (23)) found that men who consumed ten or more tomato products a week reduced their risk of aggressive prostate cancer by nearly 50 percent. If you don't like raw tomatoes, that's all right; you can flood your system with lycopene even more effectively by eating tomato products such as salsa and marinara sauce.

Blueberries owe their deep, blue color to a class of phytochemicals called **anthocyanins**. Like lycopene, anthocyanins have potent antioxidant power, but they are also true workhorses when it comes to fighting inflammation. Science is now telling us that excessive inflammation plays a major role in the development of a broad range of diseases, including heart attacks, some cancers, Alzheimer's, autoimmune disease, and allergic conditions. When you regularly consume blueberries, along with other anthocyanin rich foods, like cherries, blackberries, and raspberries, you are infusing your body with a forceful weapon against some of the most common and deadliest illnesses known to man.

Broccoli is teeming with **sulforaphane**, one of the most powerful known anticancer phytochemicals. Like lycopene and anthocyanins, this phytochemical star is also a potent antioxidant. Its special anticancer powers, though, are largely due to its ability to boost the body's detoxifying enzymes systems. Fortunately, our systems possess a remarkable class of chemicals called phase 2 enzymes. Phase 2 enzymes rid the body of carcinogens and other toxic agents. This innate system is one of the body's primary defenses against carcinogens, and it protects us from many forms of cancer, including those of the breast, lung, and colon. Eating your broccoli, along with its cruciferous cousins, cabbage, kale, cauliflower, brussels sprouts, and collards—all of which contain similar phytochemicals—will send your detoxifying, cancer-protective enzyme systems into overdrive.

Think of it this way: eating fruits and vegetables is akin to adding a turbo to a car. Fruits and vegetables supercharge the body's metabolic engine so that our natural biological processes occur faster and more efficiently than they would otherwise. This is an especially apt metaphor for all you veggie-resistant gentlemen out there—and according to the National Cancer Institute, there are quite a few of you. The NCI reports that **96 percent of the American male population does not get the recommended seven to nine servings of fruits and vegetables daily,** despite the fact that these foods lower the risk of cancer, protect against heart attacks, and prolong the male sex life. Unfortunately, men are trained to pile on the protein from an early age, and in the process, they often fail to realize that vegetables are just as integral to building muscle, strength, stamina, and strong bones as protein is.

If you are one of these veggie-challenged men, I'm here to tell you there is nothing "masculine" about artery-clogging cholesterol and saturated fat. In the current age of health consciousness, veggies (and fruit) are far sexier than a giant serving of prime rib or steak. If you need to incorporate more vegetables into your diet, here are a few snack and meal strategies for a more "manly" diet: eat sliced apples with almond butter; toss a handful of veggies in an omelet; add extra lettuce, tomatoes and onions to your sandwich; put some dried apricots in your cereal; add grilled onions and mushrooms to any chicken dish; or even better, dive into some berries and yogurt for dessert.

All the Colors of the Rainbow

Nature's storehouse is filled with delicious fruits and vegetables of almost every color and texture. From the deep blue-purple of blueberries and blackberries, to the bright orange-yellow of tangerines and bell peppers, the more colorful the food, the more packed with nutrients it is. Eat from the entire spectrum to take full advantage of the tens of thousands of beneficial compounds these foods offer. When it comes to phytochemicals, you want the entire army, not just a lone soldier. Have a little bit of every color, blue, red, green, and yellow each and every day. Remember, color means health: the deeper and richer the color, the more phytochemicals, vitamins, and minerals present in the food. Red grapefruit is always a healthier choice than white grapefruit; red onions are better than yellow onions; and deep green romaine lettuce is certainly healthier than iceberg.

A Quick Veggie Tip

Roasted vegetables are so tasty that you won't believe you're eating "diet food." This is a wonderful cooking technique that capitalizes on the scrumptious natural taste of vegetables. Virtually any vegetable can be roasted. (Remember to stay away from starchy vegetables like white potatoes, though.) Simply place your vegetables of choice on a cookie sheet, and mist them lightly with canola or olive oil sprays or toss them in a little olive oil. Season them to your preference—try a little salt, pepper, garlic, and Italian seasoning. Roast at 425 degrees for fifteen to twenty minutes or until desired. Sprinkle with a little balsamic vinegar, and dig in.

Have a Little Fruit

Fruits are filled with the same fiber, vitamins, minerals, and phytochemicals as vegetables, and while they are an essential part of your healthy weight loss plan, it may surprise you to learn that their weight loss role should be limited.

On the 10-Step Diet, you need to consume fruit in moderation. The reason is simple—fruits contain a relatively large amount of natural sugar, and your body digests them fairly rapidly, thus raising your blood sugar level. When you eat fruits, you should optimally have a little healthy protein with it to curb their potential to elevate your blood glucose level. Have your orange with a small handful of nuts, or enjoy your berries with a little cottage cheese. That said, you would never want to cut fruit from your diet entirely; like vegetables, fruits contain a stunning array of phytochemicals that can literally ward off diseases.

Everyone knows that oranges contain vitamin C and bananas contain potassium, but what you may not know is how many other disease-fighting compounds are contained in fruits. For example, the number one superstar—blueberries—contains more than a dozen vitamins and minerals, and nearly a hundred phytochemicals. An orange provides vitamin C, folate, fiber, and every known class of natural anticancer compound making them nature's perfect anticancer package.

Apples are yet another superstar food, containing a hundred and fifty health-promoting compounds. In fact, findings from Finland suggest an apple a day really may keep the doctor away. In a study of more than ten thousand men and women, those who consumed the most flavonoid phytochemicals, especially one type called quercitin that is more abundant in apples than any other fruit, were less likely to die from heart disease or develop lung cancer, asthma, or diabetes (*American Journal of Clinical Nutrition*, September 2002, Volume 76 (3)).

The Superstar Fruits for Wellness and Weight Loss

· Berries

· Pomegranates

· Cherries

· Plums

· Any whole citrus (oranges, red grapefruit, tangerines, etc.)

· Cantaloupe

· Red grapes

· Peaches

· Apples

· Pears

· Apricots—dried or fresh

Despite the powerful compounds found in fruits, **for the first week of my 10-Step Diet, I recommend that you avoid all fruits** *except* **berries.** (See Part 2.) When it comes to strawberries, blueberries, blackberries, and raspberries, I encourage you to incorporate these fruits—fresh or frozen—into your diet on a regular basis starting on day one. For those who want to improve their health and lose weight, these fruits are the *crème de la crème*: berries are naturally low in calories (less than 70 cal/cup), have a low glycemic index, taste delicious, and are brimming with some of the most powerful phytochemicals known, making them Mother Nature's preeminent antioxidants. Consider the first week of this plan your "phytochemical induction phase."

James Joseph Ph.D, professor of nutrition at Tufts University, released the first major study on the potential effects of fruits and vegetables to reverse age-related decline in brain function. According to his findings, a diet rich in blueberry extract (comparable to one cup of blueberries daily) decreased short-term memory loss and actually reversed some loss of balance and coordination in aging rats. In an earlier study by Tufts and USDA researchers, blueberries topped a list of fifty fruits and vegetables for potency of disease-fighting antioxidants.

Recently, however, another fruit superstar has come onto the scene: pomegranates. Studies suggest pomegranates could become the next "superfood" as research indicates the phytochemical profile of this fruit shows that 100 ml of pomegranate juice is two to three times richer in antioxidants than that found in 100 ml of red wine or green tea—some of the most potent antioxidants ever documented. In fact, pomegranates contain flavonoids that are even more concentrated than those found in red grapes, the current flavonoid superstar.

With the countless nutrients and health benefits, apples, oranges, berries, pomegranates, and other superstar fruits offer, we should all make an effort to eat them daily.

Berries are low in calories, high in fiber, loaded with phytochemicals, and totally adaptable—they can be eaten fresh or frozen, tossed into salads, smoothies, yogurt, cereal, cottage cheese, or eaten alone. And, if you are wondering why berries are included on the first week of the diet, to the exclusion of all other fruits, read on!

Raspberries are packed with more fiber than any other fruit. They are also an outstanding source of vitamin C and manganese, two powerful antioxidants, and contain ten other essential nutrients and phytochemicals, including ellagic acid, famous for its anti-cancer prowess.

Strawberries, the beauty queen of all the fruits, prove to be an excellent source of vitamin C. Believe it or not, strawberries contain more vitamin C than oranges. They are also good sources of folic acid and potassium, important nutrients for heart health.

Blueberries, Mother Nature's diminutive, but all-powerful fruit holds first place out of forty-nine other fruit and vegetable contenders on Tufts University's ORAC score. The ORAC score represents the measured antioxidant power of various fruits and vegetables. But it's no wonder blueberries scored so high at Tufts! They are the perfect brain food. Blueberries are not only incredibly effective antioxidants, but also powerful anti-inflammatory agents. As the brain is particularly susceptible to the destructive effects of excessive oxidation and inflammation, the unique "one-two punch" of blueberries provides powerful brain protection.

Blackberries came in a close second behind blueberries in the ORAC testing at Tufts. They, too, are an excellent source of vitamin C, potassium, and folate and abound in antioxidants, including vitamin E, ellagic acid, and anthocyanin pigments.

Step 5 Action Plan: Vegetables and Fruit

*This is the one food group I'm going to ask you to count, as it is vital to your weight loss and wellness goals to ensure you get **all** of the recommended servings.*

Vegetables
· Consume five or more servings a day.
· A serving is a half-cup raw or cooked of any vegetable *except* dark leafy greens.
· For dark leafy greens (spinach, lettuce, collards, etc.) one serving is 1 cup uncooked.
· Vegetables can be consumed fresh or frozen.
· Avoid the starchier, higher glycemic index vegetables: potatoes, parsnips, rutabagas, and corn.
· Avoid canned vegetables because of inferior nutritional quality and high sodium content with the exception of tomatoes, tomato products, roasted red peppers, and artichokes.

Fruit
· For the first week of this diet, the only fruits permitted are berries: blueberries, blackberries, raspberries, and strawberries. Limit yourself to no more than 1 cup (two servings) a day. After the first week, consume two servings of any superstar fruit a day. (Select from the above list.)
· Avoid the sweeter, higher glycemic index tropical fruits: bananas, pineapple, mangos, and papayas.
· With the exception of apricots, avoid dried fruits, as they have a very high glycemic index.
· Fruit can be consumed fresh or frozen as long as they contain no added sugar.
· Avoid canned fruit as they generally contain added sugar and are nutritionally inferior.

*When you consume your fruit, **always** have some healthy protein with it. This will minimize its potential to elevate your blood glucose level.*

EAT HIGH QUALITY PROTEIN AT EACH MEAL

Protein Secrets

Healthy forms of protein are fantastic allies in your weight loss endeavor. Contrary to refined carbs, when proteins are digested, they produce a prolonged and steady level of glucose in the blood, staving off hunger for longer periods of time. Combine proteins with carbs, and those carbs will enter your bloodstream as glucose more slowly, resulting in a reduced insulin response. Proteins delay gastric emptying, which means food stays in your stomach longer. This slows down the digestive process overall, and enhances the feeling of fullness in your stomach, which will further suppress your appetite.

Like carbohydrates, when it comes to protein and healthy weight loss, some forms of protein are better for you than others. The difference is not so much the *type* of protein, but the *package* it comes in. The healthiest protein packages are those that don't contain excessive amounts of unhealthy food components like saturated and trans fats, but rather contain other health-promoting nutrients.

Let's look at a simple example: A 6-ounce broiled Porterhouse steak is a great source of complete protein—in fact, 38 grams worth. But it also delivers 44 grams of fat, 16 grams of which are saturated—and that's almost three-fourths of the FDA recommended daily intake for saturated fat! The same portion of salmon provides 34 grams of protein, only 4 grams of saturated fat and 18 grams of mostly good fats—including omega 3, the superstar fat, which we will discuss at length in the coming pages. A cup of cooked lentils has 34 grams of protein, delivers less than 1 gram of good fat and is loaded with fiber, vitamins, minerals, and those magnificent disease-fighting phytochemicals we heard so much about in the previous step.

From this simple example we can see that there is something to be said about reducing your intake of red meat. At the moment, research on whether specific animal proteins are better or worse for you than specific vegetable proteins is incomplete; however, I recommend that you begin replacing some animal protein with vegetable protein, if only to jumpstart your weight loss and take advantage of their fiber, phytochemicals, and lack of saturated fat.

Healthy protein plays a vital role in your overall wellness and weight loss plan. These foods will not rapidly elevate your level of blood insulin; in fact, your insulin levels barely budge when protein is consumed. I recommend that you have some form of healthy protein with each and every meal—and I do mean every meal, *especially* breakfast.

"Every Meal" Means *Every Meal*

For ages now, we have all heard that breakfast is the number one
ingredient in the recipe for an energized, productive day. When it
comes to dieting, it is doubly true. By eating some healthy protein at
breakfast, you will be preparing yourself for a *successful* and *stress-
free* day of dieting. Compelling studies have shown that those who
incorporate healthy proteins into their breakfast routines will eat less
throughout that day, as opposed to folks who eat a breakfast
comprised of carbs. If you are really committed to losing weight, this
is one strategy that you must incorporate into your lifestyle; it will
increase your success rate and your vitality in general.

Omega-3 eggs are a great way to start your day on the right
foot. We will discuss the merits of omega-3 fats when we reach Step
7, but for the moment, you should know that getting as many omega-
3 fats in your diet as you can is one of the most important nutritional
strategies you can employ to promote your health. Omega 3 is a
special polyunsaturated fat, and the chickens that lay these superstar
eggs are fed a diet enriched with omega 3. These eggs are now available in almost all grocery outlets and can provide up to a hundred
times *more* omega-3 fats than the standard supermarket eggs! You
will pay a little more, but it's worth it. Look for the words "omega-
3 fatty acid," "DHA," or "EPA" (two specific forms of omega 3) to
be sure you are getting the healthiest eggs available.

Something's Fishy

Overwhelming medical data supporting why everyone should eat more fish continues to mount. Populations that eat more fish have less heart disease, less cancer, less depression, less arthritis, less impotence, and less Alzheimer's disease. Most experts agree this is likely due to the abundant omega-3 marine oils uniquely found in this food group. Oily fish (salmon, tuna, mackerel, sardines, herring, and lake trout) contain especially high amounts of omega 3, so make them your first choice. (However, please see the action plan for a word of caution about tuna and farm raised salmon.)

The Scoop on Soy

There is probably no other food that has received more spin or recent attention than soy—and rightfully so.

Soy boasts an exemplary nutritional profile—complete protein, heart-healthy omega-3 fats, vitamins, minerals, fiber, and phytochemicals. Studies have shown conclusively that regular consumption of soy foods—especially if you're eating soy to replace animal proteins high in saturated fat, such as beef and pork—lowers LDL (bad) cholesterol and offers significant cardiovascular protection. Promising scientific studies show that soy foods may also offer protection against cancer, especially the hormonally sensitive cancers—breast, ovarian, and prostate. However, I stress *may*, as definitive studies are not yet available. Still, given its highly nutritious makeup and heart-healthy benefits, soy is worthy of our attention; if you enjoy soy foods, you should strive to have several servings a week.

My Beef with Red Meat

I love red meat (beef, pork, and lamb), but I make a concerted effort to limit my indulgences to two servings or less a week. If you read what I have, I'm sure you would do the same. Many studies have revealed a strong association between heavy red meat consumption (which includes hamburgers) and deadly diseases such as heart disease, prostate cancer, and colon cancer. Here are eight specific reasons to follow my lead and curtail your intake of red meat.

1. Red meat contains lots of saturated fat. Eating excessive saturated fat can increase your risk of heart disease and promote insulin resistance.

2. Red meat is a rich food source of arachidonic acid. Arachidonic acid is an infamous fatty acid molecule from which all of the pro-inflammatory eicosanoids arise. Inflammation plays a prominent role in the pathogenesis of cardiovascular disease, Alzheimer's disease, allergies, asthma, autoimmune conditions, and some forms of cancer. Additionally, a recent landmark study published in the *New England Journal of Medicine* (January 1, 2004, Volume 350 (1)) found that one in six Americans carry a gene variant that dramatically increases their risk of heart disease, especially when food high in arachidonic acid (red meat) is consumed.

3. Standard red meat from domesticated animals contains omega-6 fatty acids and minimal to no omega-3 fatty acids. All domesticated livestock, with the exception of free range livestock, are fed artificial diets heavy in omega-6 fats from grains, corn, and soy. Excessive consumption of red meat contributes to an unhealthy omega-6: omega-3 fatty acid ratio.

4. Red meat may contain cancer causing chemicals. A potent class of known carcinogens called HCAs (heterocyclic amines) form within the protein fibers of red meat when heated at high temperatures (grilling, barbequing, and frying). A second class of carcinogens, nitrosamines, can form in the gastrointestinal tract from sodium nitrite contained in processed and cured meats (bacon, ham, salami, bologna, hot dogs, and other processed luncheon meats).

5. Red meat (especially beef) contains high concentrations of iron. Iron from red meat, unlike vegetable sources of iron, is absorbed from the gastrointestinal tract whether the body needs it or not. Excess iron in the bloodstream behaves as a potent pro-oxidant and has been implicated in promoting heart disease, breast cancer, and colon cancer.

6. Red meat contains potentially harmful "added ingredients." Virtually all domesticated livestock (with the exception of those deemed organic or free range) contain antibiotic and sex steroid hormonal residues. Excessive exposure to the former may predispose humans to resistant bacterial pathogens; excessive exposure to the latter may predispose humans to hormonally sensitive cancers: breast, prostate, and ovarian.

7. Red meat exists high on the food chain. As you move up the food chain, harmful environmental contaminants and toxins concentrate. Eating red meat that comes from the apex of the food chain increases your exposure to harmful agents such as pesticides, herbicides, heavy metals, PCBs, dioxins, and so on.

8. Red meat may contain harmful viruses and bacteria. Undercooked red meat can lead to potentially life-threatening infections.

Can You Get Too Much Protein?

Too little protein is clearly a problem. What about too much?

Protein is an essential nutrient for cell maintenance and repair as well as the regulation of a wide range of bodily functions. How much protein we need to eat in our diet depends on our age, lean body mass, activity level, and health status. The average adult female requires about 50 grams a day and the average adult male, 65 grams a day for maintenance of normal bodily functions. A cup of yogurt at breakfast (12 grams), 3 ounces of tuna at lunch (20 grams), 4 ounces of chicken at dinner (28 grams), and a 1 ounce snack of almonds (6 grams) would suffice.

Many in the medical establishment are concerned by the excessive protein intake recommended by some "no-carb" or "low-carb" diet plans, as such recommendations may have a negative impact on kidney and bone health over the long run. As a normal by-product of protein metabolism, acid is released into the bloodstream after protein is consumed. This acid has to be neutralized or buffered; as we learned in Step 3, calcium, which may be taken from bones, is used to perform this task. The kidneys then excrete these calcium-acid waste products through urine.

It is well established that high protein diets promote urinary excretion of calcium. A short-term commitment to a high protein diet is unlikely to have a significant effect on bone health, but adhering to a diet such as this for an extended period of time may very well compromise bone integrity and predispose a person to osteoporosis. In the Nurses' Health Study, women who ate more than 95 grams of protein a day were 20 percent more likely to have broken a wrist over a twelve year period, compared to those who ate an average amount of protein, less than 68 grams a day (*American Journal of Epidemiology*, March 1, 1996, Volume 143 (5)).

As already mentioned, the kidneys are responsible for releasing the acidic by-products of protein metabolism. When faced with excessive protein loads, the kidneys indeed may be overtaxed. A recent Harvard based study (*Annals of Internal Medicine*, March 18, 2003, Volume 138 (6)) found that high protein diets in women, particularly from meat, increased the rate of kidney decline in those with pre-existing mild kidney dysfunction. This was not the case for women with healthy kidneys. The elderly and people with high blood pressure, diabetes, and gout are at high risk for mild kidney dysfunction and should likely avoid long-term use of high protein diet plans.

Yogurt Cheese—A Super Healthy Mayonnaise Alternative

This extremely versatile, silky smooth "cheese" is a tasty and nutritious alternative to mayonnaise. It provides calcium, protein, B vitamins, and has fewer calories. You can use yogurt cheese instead of mayo for spreads, sauces, dips, and dressings. To make yogurt cheese, line a colander, sieve, or funnel with a coffee filter. Pour desired amount of plain, low-fat yogurt in the filter and drain in the refrigerator for five to twenty hours. The longer you drain, the thicker it becomes. After twenty hours, 2 cups of yogurt yields 1 cup yogurt cheese.

Step 6 Action Plan: Healthy Protein

- Be sure to have some healthy protein at each meal.
- Be especially vigilant in consuming protein at breakfast. Try nuts/seeds, soy milk, low-fat milk, peanut butter or other nut butters, smoked or canned salmon, low-fat yogurt, Canadian bacon, omega-3 eggs, cottage cheese, or other reduced-fat cheeses.
- Strive to have one serving (a half cup) of bean/legumes daily.
- Strive to have three servings of fish a week (preferably oily fish—see below).
- Always choose *healthy* animal proteins:
  - Oily fish: salmon, tuna, mackerel, sardines, herring, and lake trout are the best.
  - Skinless poultry: chicken and turkey.
  - Omega-3 fortified eggs.
  - Shellfish: oysters, clams, shrimp, scallops, crab, lobster, and so on.
  - Low-fat dairy products: skim or 1% milk, part-skim, or reduced-fat cheeses.
  - Wild game: venison, quail, and dove, etc.

Limit red meat (beef, pork, lamb) to two or less servings a week. When you do eat red meat, choose leaner cuts such as loin and center cuts.

Fresh tuna and canned white Albacore tuna are moderately high in methyl mercury, a heavy metal that can be toxic to the brain and kidneys. I recommend you limit fresh tuna to no more than four servings a month and choose canned chunk light tuna as an alternative to albacore.

Additionally, recent studies have revealed that farm raised salmon, may contain excessive levels of PCBs, a cancer promoting environmental contaminant. Therefore, I also recommend you limit fresh farm raised salmon (also called Atlantic salmon) to four servings a month and choose its Wild Alaskan counterpart (available canned, frozen, and occasionally fresh) as the healthier alternative.

Pregnant and nursing women, and children under six are uniquely vulnerable to the toxic effects of methyl mercury and PCBs, and should further restrict consumption of these varieties of fish.

Everyone should strictly avoid the large, carnivorous fish (marlin, shark, swordfish, tile fish, and king mackerel) because they contain high concentrations of PCBs, dioxins, and methyl mercury.

HAVE YOUR FATS AND
EAT THEM TOO

Fabulous, Fantastic Fats

Over the past few decades, fats have received a very bad rap—especially when you stop to consider the crucial role they play in keeping your body going. Believe it or not, fat is a vital structural component of all cell membranes and the lining of our nerves. Fat is required for the transport of fat-soluble vitamins and phytochemicals from our intestines to the bloodstream. Furthermore, fat plays an indispensable part in supplying the building blocks or raw materials for many hormones, including the eicosanoids, which govern all of the life processes in our bodies, from blood clotting to cellular respiration.

And let's be honest: fats add a lot of flavor to food. Fats do not elevate our blood glucose or insulin levels—a fact which is critical to weight loss and your health in general, as we discussed at length in Step 1. In fact, fats operate in ways contrary to quickly digested, white carbs; they provide a dense source of calories (9 calories/gram as opposed to 4 calories/gram in carbohydrates). As such, they are very effective appetite suppressants. Additionally, like proteins, they can slow the digestive process, keeping you feeling fuller longer.

If you still aren't convinced that some fats can be good for you, consider this: over the past forty years, Americans have decreased their consumption of daily fat calories from 40 percent to 34 percent; and yet, over this same period of time, Americans have become heavier than ever before. Meanwhile, and not surprisingly, rates of type 2 diabetes have skyrocketed, and cardiovascular disease remains our number one killer. Why?

Well, in part because "low-fat" diets that swapped a healthy egg for a bagel became all the rage. As you now know, highly refined carbohydrates, while low in fat, aren't going to help you lose weight—quite the opposite, in fact. In addition, exchanging healthy fat for refined carbs can predispose a person to insulin resistance and frequently leads to an elevation of blood triglycerides and a reduction of HDL (good) cholesterol.

There is not a shred of scientific data to support the notion that eating additional fat calories is any more fattening than eating additional carbohydrate or protein calories. As we have seen throughout the 10-Step Diet, when it comes to healthy weight loss and wellness, it is not just *quantity* that matters, but also the *quality*. When approached in an informed manner, the "right" fats provide you with yet another nutritional strategy to protect your health and help you reach and sustain your weight loss goals. In this step, therefore, we are going to talk about the fats you should include in your diet, the fats you should limit, and the fats you should avoid like the plague.

The Fat Facts

There are four categories of dietary fats found in our food supply. Two of these categories, namely saturated fat and trans fat, have no health value. To the contrary, they provide unhealthy calories you don't need and cause metabolic chaos, especially within your cardiovascular system. They are the "wrong" fats; avoid them as best you can.

On the other hand, the other categories of dietary fats, monounsaturated fats and polyunsaturated fats, can literally make you healthier. The superstar fat I have mentioned throughout this book, omega 3, is a polyunsaturated fat. Along with the monounsaturated variety, these are the "right" fats, and on the 10 Step Diet you will be able to indulge in them, enhance the flavor of your foods with them, and take advantage of their proven health benefits.

While consuming the "wrong" fats (trans fat and saturated fat) will provoke disease and may predispose you to weight gain, eating the "right" fats (monounsaturated fat and polyunsaturated fats, such as omega 3) can dramatically lower your risk of heart disease and stroke, lessen inflammation in your body, improve your neurological and mental health, and reduce your risk of insulin resistance. Of course, before we talk about the "right" fats, we need to talk about the "wrong" ones—and make sure you strip them from your lifestyle, purge them from your pantry, and keep them out of your shopping cart altogether.

The Wrong Fats: Saturated and Trans Fats

Saturated fats are primarily found in animal products: red meat, poultry skin, and whole dairy products. They are also found in tropical oils, such as coconut and palm oil. Saturated fats are the dietary culprit infamous for raising your bad cholesterol, also called LDL, which is known to be a powerful risk factor for cardiovascular disease.

Studies have shown that saturated fats can also elevate blood triglycerides (another bad fat found in the blood), increase blood platelet stickiness (a precursor to all heart attacks and most strokes), contribute to insulin resistance (the fat-loving metabolic state linked to obesity, heart disease, and type 2 diabetes), and possibly increase the risk of certain cancers.

Researchers at Johns Hopkins University report (American College of Cardiology Meeting, March 30, 2003) that people who eat a diet high in saturated fat accumulate more fat around their internal organs and in the abdomen than those who eat the healthier polyunsaturated fats. This so-called visceral fat, or abdominal obesity, is a powerful risk factor for diabetes and cardiovascular disease.

A study published in the April 2002 issue of the *Annals of Internal Medicine* (Volume 136 (7)) found that for five hours after a single high-saturated fat meal (equivalent to a fast food half-pound burger with fries), blood triglycerides (a bad blood fat) rose from 100 mg/dl to 250 mg/dl and coronary flow reserve decreased by 18 percent. When heart arteries become blocked, the blood vessels around them expand to compensate. The increased or compensated blood flow that results is the coronary flow reserve. In other words, for those with underlying heart disease (blocked arteries), a single high saturated fat meal may indeed diminish blood flow to the heart, which in some cases, may be enough to trigger a heart attack.

But if saturated fats are the great white shark, then trans fats are the killer whale. At the moment, it is estimated that the average American consumes 4-8 percent of their daily calories as trans fats—and this is 4-8 percent too much. Trans fats are the unhealthiest ingredients in our food supply, and I urge you to rid your diet of them completely. Simply open your pantry and throw out any and all products containing "trans fats." To identify these products, check food labels for "shortening," "hydrogenated oil," or "partially hydrogenated oil." Do the same when you are at the grocery store, and make a pact with yourself that trans fats will not go into your shopping cart.

Why do we need to be so vigilant when it comes to trans fat? Why are these fats so hazardous to our health?

Structurally, trans fats are a bizarre and unnatural form of fat derived from a modern food technology process called hydrogenation. During hydrogenation, liquid vegetable oils are infused with hydrogen ions to create a fat that is more solid at room temperature. Food manufacturers prefer these hydrogenated, or partially hydrogenated, oils primarily because of their longer shelf life. And unfortunately, due to the rise of prepared and processed food products, trans fats have made their way into an unbelievable number of food items we have come to know and rely on. Trans fats are found in most margarines, shortenings, and foods containing hydrogenated or partially hydrogenated oils.

These ever-present fats assault your cardiovascular system in four distinct ways: First, they elevate your LDL (bad) cholesterol. Second, they lower your HDL (good) cholesterol. Third, they increase blood platelet stickiness. And finally, they may even elevate your triglycerides. They also have been associated with breast cancer and found to increase insulin resistance.

The famous Harvard based Nurses' Health Study found that participants who took just 2 percent of their daily calories in the form of trans fat and substituted a healthier form of fat, diminished their risk of cardiovascular disease by a whopping 53 percent (*New England Journal of Medicine*, November, 20, 1997, Volume 337 (21)).

Trans Fats Unmasked

Despite the fact that trans fats are found in most processed baked goods, snack foods, and fried fast foods, you wouldn't know it by looking at the nutrition facts listed on their food labels. As a result, many Americans are consuming significantly more bad fat than they think.

The Center for Science in the Public Interest recently sent several processed foods to an independent laboratory for analysis of their trans fat content. Many foods were found to have additional grams of fat in the form of trans fat over and above the total fat grams listed on the nutritional label. Examples included a brand of potpie found to have an additional 6.5 grams of trans fat, and a frosted donut with 5 additional grams of trans fat.

Thankfully, the situation is about to get much better; the FDA now recognizes the dangers of trans fats and will require all food manufacturers to clearly label the amount of trans fat in the foods they manufacture by 2006.

Things are improving on the restaurant front also. In November 2003, Ruby Tuesday, one of the nation's largest casual dining chains, became the country's first restaurant to switch from hydrogenated oil (laden with trans fat) to heart-healthy canola oil for their frying medium. Alas, most national chains still fry in heavily hydrogenated oils.

The Right Fats: Monounsaturated and Polyunsaturated Fats

Now that we have cleared your cupboards and shopping carts of these dangerous fats, we can replace them with healthy ones.

Unlike their manmade trans fat cousins, monounsaturated fats are plant-derived fats and remain in a liquid form at room temperature. The most famous monounsaturated fat is olive oil, but canola oil, a milder oil derived from the rape plant, also belongs in this special family of fats. Avocados, which are actually fatty fruits, contain monounsaturated fats, as do many nuts and seeds.

These fats offer four impressive cardiovascular benefits—in fact, the difference between the "wrong" fats and the "right" fats is like night and day. Monounsaturated fats can lower your LDL (bad) cholesterol, decrease blood platelet stickiness (less blood clotting reduces your risk of heart attacks and strokes), decrease the chances of an erratic heartbeat (arrhythmia), and may even elevate your good (HDL) cholesterol.

If you start to include monounsaturated fats in your diet as your main fat source, you'll not only feel great about what you are doing for your body, but you'll also improve insulin sensitivity, which for many means enhanced weight loss. Furthermore, their *quadruple* cardiovascular protection will seriously reduce your chances of requiring a *quadruple bypass*. Keep this in mind each and every time you "just say no" to butter and dip your sourdough or whole grain bread in extra virgin olive oil.

The polyunsaturated fats also remain liquid at room temperature and are found in both marine and plant life. The polyunsaturated fats derived from plants (corn oil, safflower oil, sunflower oil, cottonseed oil) have been shown to lower LDL (bad) cholesterol, but lack some of the other positive health attributes of monounsaturated fats. In addition, these polyunsaturated fats are a rich source of omega-6 fats, one of the two essential fats. Unfortunately, many experts, including myself, believe the omega-6 fats have become dangerously plentiful in our diet through the preponderant use of vegetable oils in processed foods, thereby putting our health at risk. I heartily recommend that you choose canola and olive oil over these vegetable oils.

Science Made Simple—Understanding the Omega 6: Omega 3 Ratio

It is impossible to talk about the "right" fats without discussing the merits of omega-3 and omega-6 fats and taking the time to understand their relation to one another. As mentioned above, Americans currently consume an overabundance of omega-6 fats relative to omega-3 fats. In reality, these fats are designed to work together; too much of one and not enough of the other is dangerous to your health. It is extremely important, therefore, to understand the optimal ratio between the two, as it is vital to both your weight loss goals and your health in general.

Of all the functions essential fats perform in our bodies, one of the most important is providing the building blocks or raw materials for the eicosanoid class of hormones. These hormones govern virtually all of the life processes in our body, including cellular respiration, blood clotting, immune function, inflammation, and cellular growth. Although the biochemistry of eicosanoids is extremely complex, we generally know that they are derived from both omega-6 and omega-3 fats, and further, that omega-6 and omega-3 eicosanoids have complementary roles in our bodies.

Generally, the omega-6 eicosanoids are pro-inflammatory, pro-blood clotting, and pro-cellular growth. The omega-3 eicosanoids, on the other hand, oppose these effects and are anti-inflammatory, anti-blood clotting, and anti-cellular growth. Like a see-saw that moves up and down, these two varieties of hormones constantly work toward reaching equilibrium. Unfortunately, given the predominance of omega-6 fats and the dearth of omega-3 fats in our modern American diets, the scales have been tipped in a treacherous direction.

It doesn't take a great deal of imagination to realize that an overabundance of omega-6 fats relative to omega-3 fats will encourage excessive inflammation, blood clotting, and cellular growth. Thus, a diet that indulges in omega-6 fats to the exclusion of omega-3 fats put us at risk for heart disease, Alzheimer's, arthritis, autoimmune conditions, allergies, asthma, and some cancers.

Unfortunately, as a result of modern agricultural practices and food technologies, the availability of omega-3 fats in our food supply has dramatically declined over the past century. Sixty percent of the population is deficient in this essential fat and 20 percent have blood levels so low it defies detection. Meanwhile, the amount of omega-6 fats in our foods has dramatically increased.

Those scientific experts who study the diets of our Paleolithic ancestors estimate that their diets had an equal ratio of omega 6: omega 3. Current estimates of the ratio in the modern American diet range from 14-25:1, while experts estimate the ideal ratio is likely around 4:1. Compared to our ancestors, modern Americans are consuming far more omega-6 than omega-3 fats, and most of these omega-6 fats come from processed foods containing vegetable oils and livestock that are fed omega-6 laden grain, corn, and soy instead of grazing on omega-3 rich pastures of green grass. Given the reality of the modern food culture, it is vitally important to avoid the likes of corn oil, safflower oil, sunflower oil, and cottonseed oil.

The overabundance of omega-6 fats in our diets relative to omega-3 fats may be one of the most serious nutritional problems we face in this country. And yet, as grave as this situation is, it remains underrecognized. Now that you have a basic understanding of the science behind my concerns, however, I'm sure you will agree that consuming more omega-3 fats and less omega-6 fats is critical to your wellness and vitality. Furthermore, this simple step will foster the weight loss you need.

Keeping Omega-3 Fats Close to Your Mind and Heart

While monounsaturated fats like olive and canola oil are great for weight loss and guarding your health, omega-3 fats are the hands-down superstars. On the 10-Step Diet you should eat some form of omega-3 fat daily for the health of your heart and brain and to control excessive inflammation now linked to so many diseases.

Hundreds of medical studies have demonstrated the powerful cardio-protective effects of omega-3 fats for healthy individuals, as well as those who already have heart disease. A comprehensive review of medical studies on the connection between omega-3 fats and cardiovascular disease published in the American Heart Association's journal, *Circulation* (November 19, 2002, Volume 106 (121)), reported the following cardiovascular benefits from this extraordinary class of fats:

· Decreased progression of atherosclerotic plaque
· Decreased risk of arrhythmia and sudden death
· Decreased triglyceride levels
· Decreased blood clotting
· Lowered blood pressure
· Enhanced arterial health

As a physician, I have treated a multitude of patients with cardiovascular disease and can safely say that there is no pharmaceutical agent capable of providing even two of these benefits without potential side effects. Just think: you can take advantage of all these heart-healthy benefits without a prescription and at a very reasonable price. Make sure you load your shopping cart with the omega-3 fats abundant in oily fish (salmon, tuna, mackerel, herring, lake trout, sardines), and present in lesser amounts in walnuts, soybeans, flax seed, wheat germ, omega-3 fortified eggs, and small, dark leafy greens, like purslane, and spinach.

The ancient Greek philosopher and physician Hippocrates certainly knew what he was talking about when he proclaimed, "What's good for the heart is likely good for the brain." Omega 3 not only protects your heart, but also your other vital organ—the brain.

If you take a human brain and remove all of the water, about 60 percent of what's left, or the "dry weight," of the brain is actually in the form of fat. Not the fat that we are trying to lose from our hips and thighs, but rather a structural, bioactive fat that plays a fundamental role in all aspects of brain function. The type of fat that makes up the unique fatty architecture of our brains is none other than omega 3—although, in our brains it's called DHA.

As omega-3 fats dwindle from our food supply, it is far from surprising that we are experiencing a dramatic rise in mental health conditions. Inadequate dietary consumption of omega-3 fats has been scientifically linked to a long list of twenty-first century mental and neurological disorders, including depression, bipolar disorder, reduced IQ, ADD, learning disabilities, Alzheimer's disease, and other degenerative neurological conditions. It is well established that people who eat lots of fish have lower rates of depression. The residents of Japan are a brilliant example. Traditional Japanese diets contain fifteen times more omega 3 than the standard American diet. Epidemiologic studies from Japan reveal rates of depression one-tenth the rate in this country. A 1999 Harvard based study (*Archives of General Psychiatry*, May 1999, Volume 56 (5)) found that supplementing with omega-3 fats from fish oil led to significantly longer periods of remission in bipolar patients along with improvements in nearly every other psychological outcome measure. A recent British study (*British Medical Journal*, October 26, 2002, Volume 325 (7370)) found that those who ate fish at least once a week were at reduced risk of developing dementia, including Alzheimer's disease.

Step 7 Action Plan: Fabulous, Fantastic Fats

1. Strictly avoid trans fat: stick margarines, vegetable shortening, hydrogenated and partially hydrogenated oils.
2. Only buy trans fat-free margarine—many are now available and are typically more liquid at room temperature. (The label will read "contains no trans fats.")
3. Do not eat fried fast foods—fries, chicken nuggets, burgers, fish, etc.
4. Do not buy processed foods that contain shortening or hydrogenated oils. Read the list of ingredients, and do not put anything with these hidden hazards in your shopping cart.
5. Minimize your intake of saturated fat:
   · Limit beef, pork, and lamb (red meat) to two servings or less per week. Only consume the lean cuts when you do eat red meat.
   · Do not eat poultry skin. Remove it **before** cooking, or buy only skinless poultry.
   · Avoid palm and coconut oil—processed "junk foods" are typically the only place you will find them. Make sure to read the labels.
   · Avoid full-fat dairy products—whole milk, cream, butter, or full-fat cheese. Instead, have 1% or skim milk, low-fat yogurt, part-skim or reduced-fat cheeses like mozzarella, farmer's cheese, and low-fat cheddar or Swiss. Small amounts of the highly flavored cheeses like Parmesan and feta are also acceptable.
6. Consume the monounsaturated fats as your primary form of dietary fat, including:
   · Extra virgin olive oil
   · Canola oil
   · Nut/seed oils like walnut oil or sesame oil are also acceptable if called for in recipes
   · Nuts and seeds
   · Avocados

7. Include a serving of omega-3 fats in your diet daily to include:
   - Oily fish like salmon, tuna, herring, mackerel, sardines, and lake trout
   - Walnuts
   - Canola oil
   - Omega-3 fortified eggs
   - Soybeans
   - Flaxseed or wheat germ
   - Small dark, leafy greens, such as spinach and purslane

For optimal brain and heart health (and healthier weight loss), try to eat three servings or more a week of oily fish.

STEP 8

THE KEY INGREDIENT: EXERCISE

Jumpstart Your Weight Loss

Although we have covered a great deal of nutritional ground, this non-food related step might be the most important one yet. As I have said throughout this book, diets are successful when people know why they should eat certain foods and avoid others. Unfortunately, in the current age of fad diets, it has become fashionable to make a few radical changes to the standard American meal plan and be content with the resulting weight loss. Chances are, if you have been eating white carbs morning, noon, and night, you are going to drop a significant amount of weight just by avoiding them; however, the chief complaint among those on popular diets is that they lose some weight and then can't seem to lose any more, or they quickly regain lost weight when they "go off" the diet. If you want to see profound, long-lasting results and improve your wellness overall, you have to go beyond clearing certain foods from your cupboards. Avoiding the "wrong" foods is a good start—in fact, it is a *great* start—but it is only the beginning. Our bodies are suited to expend far more energy than most of us can fathom, and the more we exercise, the more weight we will lose and the more likely we will keep it off in the long run.

Assuming that you are a non-smoker, exercising regularly is the single most powerful thing you can do to protect your health. Without argument, exercise is the closest thing we have to a magic bullet for those intent on improving their health and avoiding chronic disease. Compelling research has also shown that engaging in regular exercise is one of the most reliable predictors of your chances of successful permanent weight loss. We owe the scientists and participants of the National Weight Control Registry (NWCR) for this invaluable piece of weight loss science. Founded in 1994 and with about 4,000 subjects enrolled, the NWCR is the largest ongoing study of those who have successfully maintained slimmer waistlines. The NWCR provides unprecedented dieting insight into what really works. To be eligible for the study, participants must have maintained a 30 pound weight loss for at least one year. An impressive 91 percent of NWCR participants report regular, daily exercise. On average they spend one full hour a day taking advantage of this key ingredient. Seventy-five percent of these triumphant dieters report walking as an important component of their regimens and only 9 percent report maintaining weight loss without regular physical activity. A full 89 percent of NWCR participants report **modifying both diet and activity to achieve their weight loss.** One of my biggest personal beefs with most popular diets is that they consistently place a lopsided emphasis on diet in relation to exercise. Look at the information from the NWCR and you will have to agree. The numbers speak for themselves; in order to lose weight and keep it off, you have to do more than just eat fewer calories. You have to burn calories, too.

When it comes to exercise, that which makes you *feel* good is also good for you. Exercise enhances your longevity and can protect you from all forms of cardiovascular disease. It can protect you from breast, colon, and prostate cancer, and it will improve your immune function overall. Exercise protects you against type 2 diabetes, osteoporosis, and arthritis; it improves your balance, strength, stamina, endurance, flexibility, and proprioception (your subconscious perceptions of the movement and position of your body). Daily physical activity will enhance your quality of sleep, improve your sexual function, and even stimulate your brain. And in a culture as wired and pressed for time as ours, exercise can reduce stress, anxiety, and the likelihood of depression. Regular exercise boosts self-esteem and improves the physical appearance of our bodies.

If you were lucky enough to experience the amazing benefits of regular exercise at an early age, then you are probably already hooked. If you are not an exercise junky, I hope you will become one after you read the rest of this step. Either way, the most important thing to keep in mind is it is *never* too late to benefit from the energy, vitality, joy, good health, peace of mind, and exhilaration that comes as a result of physical exercise. Daily physical exercise is a gift only you can give yourself, and it is a gift you deserve.

Taking the First Step

There are some important considerations to keep in mind when you start your exercise program. The first is to pick an activity that you truly enjoy. If you try to consistently engage in an exercise that you really don't like, the chances of doing it faithfully for the rest of your life are rather slim. If you can't stand jogging, think about riding a bicycle; if a bicycle seat bores you, consider swimming. Given the range of choices—from the variety of classes offered at your local gym, to extreme sports and that old standby, walking—rest assured, you will be able to find a sport or activity perfect for your needs.

As you embark on any of the lifestyle changes outlined in the 10 Step Diet, remember that it takes about six months for a new behavior to become internalized. Daily exercise is no different. Be patient with yourself, yet dogged in your pursuit of total wellness. In order to secure a lifetime of health, exercise has to become a planned, almost compulsive activity just like brushing your teeth. There will be days when excuses will seem justified, but when it comes to your health, "I don't have time," is a feeble rationalization. Your health is something for which you have to *make* the time, and committing 2 percent of your day—just a mere thirty minutes—is all it takes to reap the rewards.

My Personal Exercise Experience

I first experienced the virtues of regular exercise as a teenager and have been hooked ever since. If it weren't for my daily exercise regime, I don't think I would be half the person I am today. On countless occasions exercise has:

· Lifted my mood

· Empowered me to muster up the courage and perseverance to accomplish things I never thought possible

· Relieved my anxiety

· Dissipated my anger

· Dried my tears

· Revitalized my tired body

· Provided the solitude necessary to solve and reconcile difficult personal issues

· Invigorated my brain and provided me with clarity of thought

---

If the thought of exercising at least thirty minutes a day seems overwhelming, remember that there is no shame in starting small. Even tri-athletes begin somewhere.

If it has been some time since you last engaged in planned exercise, consider wearing a pedometer. A pedometer will provide you with an assessable gauge to measure your daily activity. For people who lead sedentary lives, studies have shown that using a pedometer and meeting a daily quota of steps is a great way to reduce body fat and see quantifiable improvements in fitness levels. Remember that any time you walk, those steps count—whether it's around the block, or just to and from the living room.

Take a baseline of how many steps you take each day and then make it your goal to take additional steps thereafter. If you're more sedentary than active, you'll probably find that you average two to four thousand steps daily. According to a Harris poll, the average American walks 5,310 steps in a day; unfortunately, this is only half of what is needed to maintain good fitness levels. Once you have an understanding of your current activity, you can start adding another thousand steps each day, with an ultimate goal of taking ten thousand steps or more before you get into bed each night. It might sound like a lot, but ten thousand steps is the recommended daily average for a healthy lifestyle. Keep in mind that a ten minute walk will add about a thousand steps to your daily count.

For the majority of people, walking is the perfect form of exercise: our bodies are specifically designed to walk, it's free, and you can do it anywhere. Furthermore, walking actually exercises more than just your physical body; it exercises your brain, too. Walking requires a skill known as cross-patterned movement. With each stride, one leg and the opposite arm move forward simultaneously; for example, right arm, left leg. The movement is then repeated with the opposite limbs in the next stride. While it sounds awfully simple, the movement is quite complex. In fact, cross-patterned movement generates electrical activity in your brain known to have harmonious effects on your entire central nervous system.

Energize Your Body

Not unlike a great many other human endeavors, exercise has cumulative results. If you dedicate a half hour of your day to walking 2 miles, which burns about 200 calories, and keep your caloric intake in check, you can lose an additional half pound a week. Cumulatively, this adds up to 22 pounds annually.

Regular exercise doesn't just help you burn calories while you're sweating away on the Stairmaster, though; because exercise increases your lean body mass (your muscles), it also increases your metabolism. Your resting metabolic rate—the amount of calories you burn while sedentary—is largely determined by your lean body mass. The more you exercise, the more lean body mass you have, and the higher your resting metabolic rate becomes. If you want to lose weight, you want all the muscle you can get; if you exercise regularly, your body's metabolism increases, and you will burn more calories when you are at rest than you would if you did not engage in exercise at all.

Exercise also lowers and stabilizes blood glucose and insulin levels. Muscle cells are loaded with insulin and glucose receptors, and when used, they are remarkably effective in extracting glucose and insulin from the bloodstream. For those with insulin resistance and the excess blood insulin levels accompanying this condition, the remedy is regular exercise and building your lean body mass. When teamed with dietary modifications, regular exercise is an unparalleled means to overcoming insulin resistance syndrome and shedding the obstinate pounds that frequently accompany it.

Unfortunately, after the age of forty, we are preprogrammed to lose muscle fibers at a steady rate unless they are regularly called on to perform. This is the reason that the average sedentary individual's resting metabolic rate declines 10 percent per decade after the age of forty. The real "Fountain of Youth" is found in thirty minutes or more of daily moderate physical activity.

What Is Moderate Physical Activity?

The great news is that scientific studies have proven the modern adage, "no pain no gain," to be a myth. Moderately intense activity, like a brisk walk, can supply you with the same health benefits as more intense forms of exercise.

Moderate physical activity is equivalent to burning approximately 150 calories a day, or about 1,000 calories a week. Getting a moderate amount of exercise doesn't have to be a drudge. In fact, you can easily build it into your everyday life. Climb the stairs instead of using the elevator. Park your car on the opposite side of the parking lot and walk farther than usual. Pick up the pace of your yard or housework. You may not think it, but this type of "lifestyle exercise" can significantly contribute to the number of calories you burn daily. According to the National Heart, Lung and Blood Institute, common examples of moderate activity are:

· Washing and waxing a car, 45-60 minutes
· Washing windows, 45-60 minutes
· Gardening, 35-40 minutes
· Pushing a stroller 1-1½ miles in 30 minutes
· Raking leaves, 30 minutes
· Walking 2 miles in 30 minutes
· Shoveling snow, 15 minutes
· Stair walking, 15 minutes

- Playing volleyball, 45-60 minutes
- Shooting baskets, 30 minutes
- Swimming laps, 30 minutes
- Jumping rope, 15 minutes
- Bicycling 5 miles in 30 minutes
- Water aerobics, 30 minutes

Staying Motivated

On days that you can't bear the thought of exercise, commit to taking the first few steps. You will almost always go ahead and finish the entire workout and feel that much more accomplished and energized for doing so. Exercise to your favorite music; studies show that when people listen to music while exercising, they actually work harder without even realizing it. Put it on your calendar and go for a walk at the same time every day. Choose interesting, beautiful places to walk, such as a zoo or a hiking trail. Turn your daily exercise time into a social event; gather some of your friends to walk with you. Or, use these thirty minutes as private, solitary time for your own reflection. Although routines are useful in establishing habitual behaviors like daily exercise, don't let your exercise program get monotonous. Keep things fresh by varying your workouts; bike one day, jog the next, and swim on another.

For weight loss purposes, early morning is the ideal time to exercise. After an overnight fast, your blood and body glucose stores are at their lowest; this means that you will have a greater chance of using and burning your fat stores. If early morning exercise is impossible, don't eat for several hours before your workout. In my experience, those who habitually exercise in the early morning or during lunchtime have the greatest success with incorporating exercise as a daily and long-term endeavor.

Step 8 Action Plan: Exercise

The perfect exercise program is the one that you can do consistently for the rest of your life. Design a program you like; make sure it includes thirty minutes or more of moderate aerobic activity five or more days a week, fifteen to twenty minutes or more of resistance exercise (strength training) two to three days a week, and appropriate stretching.

1. Aerobic activities include: walking, running, cycling, swimming, use of fitness facility cardio machines, and organized sports like basketball, soccer, tennis, and racquetball.

2. Resistance, or strength-building activities, can be done with weight machines, free weights, Pilates, yoga, or working with elastic bands. Strength training is especially beneficial for those at risk for osteoporosis and those with insulin resistance.

3. Two to three minutes of gentle stretching *after* exercise helps maintain flexibility and good posture, while reducing the risk of injury.

Consult with your healthcare provider for an appropriate physical evaluation prior to embarking on any exercise regimen.

GO NUTS!

Indulge Your Taste Buds

Until recently, the nut might have been the most misunderstood food in America. For years, people have thought of nuts as "too fattening," when in reality, they are sources of the "right fats" (healthy monounsaturated and polyunsaturated fats, including omega-3 fats), which can ward off diseases and keep your hunger at bay.

When it comes to health-promoting performance, nuts score a perfect ten. They are healthy vegetable proteins, offering a rich supply of minerals, including zinc, copper, magnesium, boron, manganese, selenium, phosphorus, calcium, potassium, and iron. Nuts contain all forms of the antioxidant superstar vitamin E and are wonderful sources of fiber and B vitamins like thiamine, niacin, folate, and B6. They also contain antioxidant phytochemicals like that other tremendous food group, fruits and vegetables, along with phytosterols, well known for their ability to lower cholesterol.

Finally, nuts provide us with a superb source of the amino acid, arginine, which supplies the building block for the production of nitric oxide—the most important vasodilator (artery opener) in the body. Nitric oxide allows constricted arteries to relax in order to increase blood flow, along with decreasing the clotting tendency of the blood.

On top of all this, when consumed in moderation, nuts may actually help people lose weight. In a study published in the November 2003 issue of the *International Journal of Obesity* (Volume 27 (1)), participants were placed on a daily liquid diet of 1,000 calories, along with 3 ounces of almonds (384 additional calories) A second group was placed on the same 1,000 calories per day, but instead received an additional 384 calories of mixed complex carbohydrates, such as potatoes and air-popped popcorn. After twenty-four months, the almond group experienced a 62 percent greater reduction in weight/BMI, a 50 percent greater reduction in waist circumference, and a 50 percent greater reduction in fat mass as compared to the non-almond group.

Do nuts contain some special fat-melting ingredient? Likely not, but they do offer that terrific trio of fat, fiber, and protein, which effectively satisfies your appetite and keeps you feeling fuller longer. Keep a big canister of mixed nuts out on the counter and get into it whenever you feel those between-meal cravings set in. Toss them into green salads. Keep a backup stash in your pocketbook or your desk at work, and always have a generous handful a few hours before dinner. If you are like me, by the time supper is served, you will end up eating at least one-third less food than you would otherwise.

Seeds Aren't Just for the Birds

Like nuts, seeds provide a similar package of health-promoting nutrients. Pumpkin seeds, sunflower seeds, sesame seeds, and flax seeds are popular favorites perfect for the 10-Step Diet. You can incorporate seeds into almost any meal to enhance its flavor, or you can eat them on their own as a tasty snack.

Although all nuts and seeds clearly qualify for nutritional superstar status, it is interesting to note that some of them claim unique health-related features.

Brazil nuts contain more of the antioxidant mineral, selenium, than any other food. Just one **Brazil nut** supplies 140 micrograms of this important mineral, which is *two times* more than the U.S. recommended daily allowance. Adequate intakes of this trace mineral appear to play an essential role in cancer prevention. Meanwhile, **pumpkin seeds** are great sources of zinc, a nutrient deficient in many people and essential for healthy immune function. **Sunflower seeds** prove to be high in vitamin E, as well as the phyto-chemical, phenolic acid—both powerful antioxidants. **Walnuts** are the richest nut source of omega-3 fats. My favorite, the **almond**, is high in gamma tocopherol, a form of vitamin E thought to play an important role in preventing cancer and protecting your heart. **Flax seeds** are one of the most unique foods we know; they are the richest vegetable sources of omega-3 fats, with an omega 6 to omega 3 ratio of 1:3.5.

Just as nuts and seeds are dense in nutrients, they are also dense in calories, and unfortunately, calories—even in this case—do count. **Eat nuts daily, but limit your consumption to no more than 1¹/₂ ounces a day (roughly one healthy handful); see the Action Plan below for more exact measures.** This is a generous amount, more than enough to ensure that you will receive all the health and diet related benefits from these miraculous foods.

Nuts for Health

Heart disease causes an estimated 950,000 American deaths each year. Imagine if we could reduce the risk for heart disease by 30 percent—a staggering 285,000 lives could be saved annually. The cost of heart disease is almost as shocking; according to the U.S. Department of Health and Human Services our nation spends approximately 300 billion dollars every year on cardiovascular disease, which includes health expenditures plus lost productivity. Reducing heart disease just by 30 percent would cut the nation's healthcare costs by an incredible 90 billion dollars a year.

Nuts could prove to be a useful defense against the devastating effects of this widespread disease—they are virtual cardiac miracle pills. Of the eight specific attributes that make up their exemplary nutritional profile, seven of them provide documented cardiovascular protection. Several large studies have shown that consuming a small handful (1-1.5 ounces) of nuts regularly (five or more days a week) can reduce the risk of heart disease by a whopping 30-50 percent. At least eighteen clinical studies have found that adding nuts to a diet reduced in saturated fat lowers LDL (bad) cholesterol.

Additionally, California's Loma Linda University (The Seventh Day Adventist Study) studied 31,208 people and declared that **nuts are the number one food for prevention of heart attacks.** Further, study participants who ate the most nuts had less obesity than those who consumed the least nuts.

Harvard's Nurses' Health Study (*Journal of the American Medical Association*, November 27, 2002, Volume 288 (20)) found that women who consumed an ounce of nuts at least five times weekly had a 27 percent lower risk of developing diabetes compared to those who rarely ate nuts. Another study, published in the December 2003 *Archives of Ophthalmology* (Volume 121 (12)), found that consuming nuts as little as once a week reduced the risk of age-related macular degeneration (AMD) by about 40 percent. This is fantastic news, as AMD is the number one cause of adult blindness in our country.

Dr. Ann's Pumpkin Seeds Tip

One of my favorite snacks is toasted pumpkin seeds. I'm always amazed by how few people have tried this delicious and super nutritious snack. These days, you can buy fresh pumpkin seeds in bulk at most grocery stores. (Note: the seeds will be green.) Simply lay them on a baking sheet, mist lightly with canola oil, and salt lightly if desired. (The canola spray helps the salt stick to the seeds.) Roast for a few minutes at about 425 degrees, or until golden brown. Toasted pumpkin seeds make a great, wholesome snack for your entire family.

Step 9 Action Plan: Nutty Action

1. Consume nuts and seeds daily—Brazil nuts, hazel nuts, almonds, pecans, walnuts, pistachios, pine nuts, macadamias, cashews, pumpkin seeds, flaxseeds, sesame seeds, and sunflower seeds.

2. Enjoy your favorites, but strive for variety to take advantage of the full spectrum of nutrients nuts and seeds offer.

3. Use them to enhance the flavor and texture of your meals by adding them to your salads, stews, soups, sauces, etc.

4. Eat nuts as between-meal snacks. Remember, nuts and seeds are my top-rated snack for people who need to lose weight.

5. Limit your intake to no more than $1^1/2$ ounces a day. Here is a reasonably accurate count of how many nuts and seeds make up 1 ounce:
   - 18 Cashews
   - 30 Mixed nuts with peanuts
   - 24 Almonds
   - 30 Peanuts
   - 20 Hazelnuts
   - 8 Brazil nuts
   - 10 Walnuts
   - 18 Pecans
   - $1/4$ Cup sunflower seeds
   - 45 Pistachios
   - 150 Pine nuts
   - 10 Macadamias

Note: Peanuts are not actually nuts, but legumes, like peas and beans. Nutritionally, though, they are similar to tree nuts and appear to have many of the same healthful properties.

STEP 10

CONTROLLED GRAZING

Avoiding the Dieter's Downfall

Getting overly hungry is the downfall of dieters everywhere. You know how it works: you think you're behaving yourself by not eating, but you go too long between meals, and as a result, you grow so hungry that you feel as though your stomach has become a bottomless pit. While you know you should chop up some raw veggies, that box of cookies seems a whole lot closer. You grab the cookies to quell the grumbling in your stomach and promise yourself you'll be better "next time."

It's important to understand this key concept: it takes fewer food calories to *prevent* hunger, than it does to deal with it once it occurs. In addition, studies have shown that blood glucose and insulin levels remain lower and steadier over the course of the day when a given amount of food is consumed in four to five smaller, frequent feedings, as opposed to two or three larger meals. In other words, what I call "controlled grazing" is not only permitted, but also encouraged on the 10-Step Diet.

For most of us, hunger is an extremely uncomfortable state that sets us up for dietary indiscretions and overconsumption of food. Even in the rush of everyday life, we need to make time for healthy snacks. Planning ahead to keep hunger at bay is a critical strategy for successful weight loss, and part of the reason I have saved this step for last. Successful dieting requires you to understand how your body processes the food you eat. Now that you have a thorough understanding of the way different foods affect your body, you will be able to incorporate smart snacking strategies to take advantage of this knowledge and accomplish your weight loss goal.

For example, think back to the last step; you now know that nuts provide you with a dense source of healthy calories that your body will process over time, and therefore, keep you feeling fuller longer. Similarly, you know that a handful of pretzels won't have the same effect on your body; because they are made up of white carbs, your body will break them down and process them quickly—and you will be hungry again before you know it.

The same thing is true for other "fat-free" snacks like bagels and rice cakes. To keep your energy level optimal and your brain's cookie monster silent, simply choose snacks that fit the 10-Step profile, namely superstar vegetables (red pepper strips), fruit with protein (apple slices with peanut butter), whole grains with protein (AK MAK crackers with part-skim mozzarella cheese), healthy fats (avocado slices), and healthy proteins (hard-boiled eggs).

On the 10-Step Diet, you are required to eat three meals daily and snacks between those meals as necessary to maintain a state of comfortable satiety. As we discussed in Step 6 (High Quality Protein), breakfast is the most critical meal for reining in your appetite—not to mention the positive effects breakfast has on your general vitality and well-being. For reasons that have not been fully elucidated, an early morning meal following the "fasting period" of nightly sleep plays a fundamental role in controlling your appetite and reducing the chances of overconsumption later in the day, especially when that meal is rich in protein.

A study published in the *American Journal of Epidemiology* (July 1, 2003, Volume 158 (1)), which followed the eating patterns of 499 people over a one year period, found study participants who regularly skipped breakfast had 4.5 times the risk of obesity. In addition, study subjects who ate four or more times a day were 35 percent less likely to be overweight then those who ate three times a day or less. A second study presented at the American Heart Association's 43rd Annual Conference on Cardiovascular Prevention drives this point home. This study found that those who ate breakfast only twice a week or less had a 35-50 percent greater chance of developing obesity and insulin resistance syndrome than those who ate breakfast daily. Remember that insulin resistance syndrome is the precursor to all cases of type 2 diabetes and many cases of cardiovascular disease.

It is also worth noting that, for most people, metabolic rates (calorie burning potential) peak at around noon and drop thereafter. Take advantage of this by consuming a significant portion of your daily calories in the first half of the day. Along the same lines, don't eat three hours prior to bed. At the end of the day, most of us are relatively inactive, so food consumed during late night hours has a greater propensity to be stored as fat during sleep. I also recommend that you strive to eat every three to four hours. Here is a suggested meal schedule:
- Breakfast at 7:00 AM
- Snack at 10:00 AM
- Lunch at 1:00 PM
- Snack at 4:00 PM
- Dinner at 7:00 PM

Between-meal snacking will be required for most, if not all, people on this plan. One of the biggest misconceptions about dieting is that you should expect hunger. It is just not so. Hunger leads to bingeing and cravings, exactly what you *don't* need when trying to lose weight. When you trade your unhealthy eating habits for healthy ones, you'll fill your stomach with foods that won't allow you to feel hungry, and the sensation of a full stomach is your best insurance against dieting calamities. If you're looking for a healthy snack to keep hunger at bay, try some of my personal favorites:

· Dill pickles
· Canned roasted red peppers
· Cut fresh veggies like carrots, celery, bell peppers, broccoli, cauliflower, and so on. Dip them in hummus, guacamole, salsa, or olive oil and vinegar.
· Low-fat yogurt. Plain is best, but add a touch of sugar or dietetic sweetener if you must have that sweet taste.
· Nuts, of course!
· Fresh or frozen fruit. Choose from the superstar fruit discussed in Step 5, and avoid those sugary tropical fruits. Remember to always combine fruit with some form of protein, like nuts, cheese, or peanut butter to lower its potential to elevate your glucose and insulin levels.
· Soy nuts
· Dried peas with wasabi
· Part-skim mozzarella or farmer's cheese. Cheese sticks are especially convenient.
· Reduced-fat (2% milk) cheddar or Swiss cheese.
· Fruit smoothies made with skim milk, low-fat yogurt, or soy milk.
· Beef, pork, or turkey jerky
· Wasa or AK MAK crackers with cheese, almond or peanut butter, hummus, salsa, guacamole, sardines, or smoked salmon.
· Dried apricots (with nuts, cheese, or another form of healthy protein).
· Whole grain tortilla chips, dipped in hummus, salsa, or guacamole.

Dr. Ann's "Head-off-hunger-at-the-pass" Tip:

When you get home from the grocery store, take ten minutes to wash, cut, and zip several servings of raw vegetables into baggies so they're easy to grab out of the fridge when you need them for a snack.

Step 10 Action Plan: Controlled Grazing

To lose weight, eat often, using these guidelines:

1. You *must* always eat breakfast and be sure to include healthy protein at this feeding.
2. Eat a healthy lunch and dinner. Follow the suggested timeline discussed in this chapter.
3. Consume between-meal snacks as your hunger dictates.
4. Remember, small, frequent feedings are best.

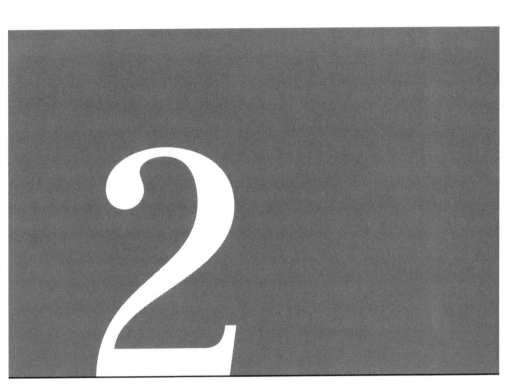

Part 2
Taking the 10 Steps

HOW TO APPROACH THIS DIET

How much weight you lose on the 10-Step Diet largely depends on how quickly you incorporate all of the steps into your daily life. Typically, I encourage my clients to implement all 10 Steps in one fell swoop; if this seems overwhelming, however, there is no shame in setting some manageable goals for yourself. That said, I want to make sure you do not misinterpret the inherent freedom of this plan: the sooner you embrace each of these steps, the sooner you will lose weight and start living a healthier and more energetic life. You deserve nothing less.

I rarely meet a person who does not already abide by at least one or two of these steps. Still, it is important to determine where *you* will need to make your biggest efforts. Ask yourself which of these steps is going to be the hardest to incorporate, and begin there. If you can't imagine a day without a soda, stop drinking it immediately; if you think exercising is for the birds, put this book down and go for a walk. If potatoes happen to be your favorite food, then begin to think about what side dishes you can have in their place. Identify the modifications that you are most anxious about and meet those challenges head on. This initiative will make following the rest of the diet much easier.

If you have been diagnosed with a medical condition or if you are at an increased risk of chronic disease, please see Part 3 for preventative measures you can take to further customize this diet to your specific health needs. Above all, remember the 10-Step Diet is *your* plan. Just as no one else can lose the weight for you, no one will be as vigilant about your wellness as you can and should be.

Unlike other diets you may have tried, the 10-Step Diet does not include a "week-by-week" guide. When it comes to changing the way you live, a week-by-week guide will only get you so far. Too many people begin a diet and falter midway because the plan is either too restrictive in its meal options or too difficult to follow. This is not true of the 10-Step Diet. While I include sample recipes and meal suggestions in Part 4, the goal of this program is to impart the wisdom that will allow you to alter your favorite dishes to fit the guidelines established here. Furthermore, with the exception of abstaining from all fruits other than berries for the first week, there are no weekly stipulations.

Take the 10 Steps

Step 1: Avoid White Carbs
Rid your diet of the "wrong carbs." Avoid white flour products, white rice, white potatoes, and sugar/sweets.

Step 2: Eat the Right Carbs
Indulge in miracle beans and great grains.

Step 3: Dump the Liquid Calories
Pour those sugar-fortified drinks down the drain, and stay away from fruit juice.

Step 4: Control Your Portions
Understand and be mindful of portion and serving sizes.

Step 5: Load Up on Veggies (And Have a Little Fruit, Too)

Have five servings of vegetables and two servings of fruit per day.

Step 6: Eat High Quality Protein at Each Meal

Limit red meat to two servings per week; choose seafood (oily fish is best), skinless poultry, beans, omega-3 eggs, low-fat dairy products, soy, and lean cuts of beef and pork.

Step 7: Have Your Fats and Eat Them Too

Avoid the "wrong" fats (saturated and trans fat), and indulge in the "right" fats (monounsaturated fats and omega-3 fats).

Step 8: The Key Ingredient: Exercise

Commit at least thirty minutes of your day to moderate physical exercise. If you can do more than that, go for it!

Step 9: Go Nuts!

Eat a variety of nuts every day; but do so in moderation— even healthy calories count.

Step 10: Controlled Grazing

Always eat breakfast, lunch, and dinner, and enjoy healthy snacks between meals.

GEARING UP FOR YOUR FIRST SHOPPING ADVENTURE

The prospect of knowing exactly what to buy for your new eating plan can be daunting. In my practice I've found that my clients' success dramatically improves when I take them through the grocery store and show them what to look for in the foods they select. I call this service my "grocery clinic."

Consider this chapter *your* grocery clinic; take this information with you the first few times you go shopping. Follow the ground rules, and use the shopping lists provided below to ensure you are stocking up on the right foods and avoiding the wrong ones. Remember, if you don't put unhealthy, forbidden foods in your grocery cart, there is no way they can make it into your cupboard.

Making Sense of Food Labels

Scrutinizing the ingredients list is far more productive then trying to decipher the nutritional table. All food manufacturers are required by law to list every ingredient in order of its quantity. By now you know there are some ingredients you should avoid, as they are known to contribute to poor health; likewise, you want to ensure you are buying the healthy foods, like whole grains. Scanning the ingredient list is usually the only way you will know what is present in that product. Because most of the foods recommended on this plan are true "whole foods," you will generally only need to refer to the nutritional labels when purchasing grain products and foods containing added sugars; the trick is to always look for more fiber and less sugar.

Commit these ingredients to memory and avoid them at all costs: trans fats (found as hydrogenated or partially hydrogenated oil and shortening), high fructose corn syrup, tropical oils (palm and coconut), refined grains (enriched wheat flour or any other grain without the word "whole" in front of it or "bran" after it), and sugar (if listed on the nutritional label as more than 10 grams).

A

Nutrition Facts
Serving Size 1 Cup (32g/1.1oz.)
Servings Per Container About 10

Amount Per Serving	Cereal	Cereal with 1/2 Cup Vitamins A&D Fat Free Milk
Calories	120	160
Calories from Fat	10	10

	% Daily Value**	
Total Fat 1g*	2%	2%
Saturated Fat 0.5g	3%	3%
Cholesterol 0mg	0%	0%
Sodium 150mg	6%	9%
Potassium 35mg	1%	7%
Total Carbohydrate 28g	9%	11%
Dietary Fiber 1g	4%	4%
Sugars 15g		
Other Carbohydrate 12g		
Protein 1g		

Vitamin A	10%	15%
Vitamin C	25%	25%
Calcium	0%	15%
Iron	25%	25%
Vitamin D	10%	25%
Thiamin	25%	30%
Riboflavin	25%	35%
Niacin	25%	25%
Vitamin B6	25%	25%
Folic Acid	25%	25%
Vitamin B12	25%	35%
Phosphorus	2%	15%
Zinc	10%	15%

* Amount in cereal. One half cup of fat free milk contributes an additional 40 calories, 65mg sodium, 6g total carbohydrate (6g sugars), and 4g protein.
** Percent Daily Values are based on a 2,000 calorie diet. Your daily values may be higher or lower depending on your calorie needs:

	Calories	2,000	2,500
Total Fat	Less than	65g	80g
Sat. Fat	Less than	20g	25g
Cholesterol	Less than	300mg	300mg
Sodium	Less than	2,400mg	2,400mg
Potassium		3,500mg	3,500mg
Total Carbohydrate		300g	375g
Dietary Fiber		25g	30g
Calories per gram: Fat 9 • Carbohydrate 4 • Protein 4			

Ingredients: Corn, wheat, and oat flour; sugar; partially hydrogenated vegetable oil (one or more of: coconut, cottonseed, and soybean); salt; sodium ascorbate and ascorbic acid (vitamin C); yellow #6; niacinamide; reduced iron; natural orange, lemon, cherry, raspberry, blueberry, lime, and other natural flavors; red #40; blue #2; zinc oxide; turmeric color; pyridoxine hydrochloride (vitamin B6); blue #1; riboflavin (vitamin B2); thiamin hydrochloride (vitamin B1); annatto color; vitamin A palmitate; BHT (preservative); folic acid; vitamin B12; vitamin D.

CONTAINS WHEAT INGREDIENTS. CORN USED IN THIS PRODUCT CONTAINS TRACES OF SOYBEANS.

Exchange: 2 Carbohydrates
The dietary exchanges are based on the Exchange Lists for Meal Planning, ©2003 by The American Diabetes Association, Inc. and The American Dietetic Association.

B

Nutrition Facts
Serving Size 1/2 cup (58 g/2oz)
Servings per Package About 10

Amount Per Serving

Calories 210	Calories from Fat 15

	% Daily Value**
Total Fat 1.5g*	2%
Saturated Fat 0g	0%
Cholesterol 0mg	0%
Sodium 260mg	11%
Total Carbohydrate 47g	16%
Dietary Fiber 7g	27%
Soluble Fiber 1g	
Insoluble Fiber 6g	
Sugars 3g	
Other Carbohydrate 37g	
Protein 7g	

Vitamin A 0%	Vitamin C 0%
Calcium 2%	Iron 8%
Phosphorus 15%	Magnesium 10%

*Amount in cereal. One half cup of fat free milk contributes an additional 40 calories, 65 mg sodium, 6 g total carbohydrate (6 g sugars), and 4 g protein.
**Percent Daily Values are based on a 2,000 calorie diet. Your daily values may be higher or lower depending on your calorie needs:

	Calories	2,000	2,500
Total Fat	Less than	65 g	80 g
Sat. Fat	Less than	20 g	25 g
Cholesterol	Less than	300 mg	300 mg
Sodium	Less than	2,400 mg	2,400 mg
Total Carbohydrate		300g	375g
Dietary Fiber		25g	30 g
Protein		50g	65g

Calories per gram:
Fat 9 • Carbohydrate 4 • Protein 4

Ingredients: Unbleached Whole Wheat Flour, Kashi® Seven Whole Grains & Sesame Flour (Stone Ground Whole: Oats, Hard Red Winter Wheat, Rye, Long Grain Brown Rice, Triticale, Buckwheat, Barley, Sesame Seeds), Malted Barley, Salt, Yeast, Mixed Tocopherols (Natural Vitamin E) for Freshness.

CONTAINS WHEAT INGREDIENTS.

To further clarify how to decipher food labels, note the two examples to the left. Included are labels for two different brands of breakfast cereal. First, refer to the ingredients list for Label A and note the first three ingredients: corn, wheat, oat flour. Because you don't see the word "whole" before any of these grains, you know you are getting refined (white) flour, which is essentially flour without fiber. Compare that to **Label B,** which lists "whole wheat flour" and seven other "whole" grains. There are no refined grains listed on **Label B,** only true whole grains.

Next, note the "hydrogenated vegetable oil," a forbidden food ingredient, listed on **Label A.** This one ingredient should be enough for you put this box of cereal right back on the shelf. In contrast, there are no hydrogenated oils listed on **Label B.**

Label A also lists "sugar" as the second most abundant ingredient in the cereal. However, you don't see any "added sugar" on **Label B.** Along with completely refined flour, sugar, and hydrogenated oil, **Label A** also includes four different chemical food colorings. Although they may not be "bad" for you, they are certainly not healthy either.

Now refer to the nutrition table. Look specifically at the fiber and the sugar content of both. Remember, fiber is good; the more the better. I recommend cereals with 5 or more grams of fiber per serving. Of course, you also need to remember that sugar is bad; the less of it, the better. I recommend avoiding products with 10 or more grams of added sugar. **Label A** lists 1 gram of fiber, whereas **Label B** list 7 grams of fiber. Additionally, **Label A** contains 15 grams of sugar, while **Label B** contains only 3 grams of sugar.

Scrutinizing the ingredients list, as well as the sugar and fiber content, provides a poignant illustration of the differences between a true wholesome food and one that is virtually 100 percent processed.

The next three or four times you go to the grocery store your shopping will likely take longer than usual; however, after a few trips, you will be a regular 10 Step master, knowing the permissible products from their imposters without even having to think about it.

Fresh Produce

Ground Rules:

Your refrigerator should be brimming with fruits and vegetables to ensure that you consume seven or more servings a day. Buy a variety, and go for color, quantity, and convenience.

Take advantage of the remarkable nutrients associated with the varied colors of fruits and vegetables. Remember, the more colorful the produce, the more phytochemicals it contains. In practical application, purple onions are better than yellow; red grapes are better than green. Red grapefruit is better than white grapefruit; winter squash, better than summer squash and so on.

Concentrate on buying the superstar fruits and vegetables listed below. Purchase convenient items in ready-to-eat bags to ensure success. Keep two or three bags of these user-friendly items (spinach, salad greens, and carrots, for example) in your refrigerator at all times. If you can afford organic, buy organic; however, know that it will spoil more quickly. Keep an eye out for the newest superstar, BroccoSprouts, which contains twenty times the cancer-fighting agent (sulforaphane glucosinolate) as whole broccoli.

THE RIGHT PRODUCE	THE WRONG PRODUCE
Superstar Cruciferous Vegetables: broccoli, cabbage, kale, collards, cauliflower, brussels sprouts, BroccoSprouts, and watercress. **Superstar Dark Leafy Greens:** spinach, darker lettuces, arugula, and purslane. **Superstars in General:** carrots, tomatoes, asparagus, garlic, onions, leeks, and red, yellow, and orange bell peppers. **Superstar Fruits:** any type of berry, pomegranates, cherries, plums, dried or fresh apricots, pears, apples, and red grapes. Any whole citrus and cantaloupe. **Superstar Apples:** Granny Smith, McIntosh, Pink Lady, and Cameo. (The tarter the apple, the lower the glycemic index.) **Bulk Raw Nuts:** Generally found in the produce section, this is the most economical way to buy them. **Fresh Herbs:** parsley, basil, dill, cilantro, chives, tarragon, oregano, etc.	**Starchy Vegetables:** potatoes, parsnips, rutabagas, and corn. **Tropical Fruits:** bananas, pineapples, mangos, and papayas. **Canned Fruits:** They are usually preserved in sugars.

Seafood, Poultry and Meat

Ground Rules:

Minimize saturated fat and maximize omega-3 fats. Opt for fresh or frozen fish, especially oily varieties due to their high omega-3 fat content. Look for fresh or frozen wild salmon (Alaskan, Pacific) fillets. Avoid the larger, carnivorous fish containing high concentrations of environmental contaminants like PCBs, dioxins, and methyl mercury.

Make every effort to buy skinless poultry, either fresh or frozen. If you buy poultry with skin, you must remove the skin before cooking. Prepackaged chicken, turkey, and ham luncheon meats are allowed. Consider using ground turkey *breast* as a substitute for ground beef. If you are a bacon lover, Canadian bacon is the best choice; turkey bacon is your second-best choice, and center cut, or reduced-fat bacon, is your third choice. When choosing beef or pork, go for the lean cuts. Wild game, if available, is also an excellent choice.

THE RIGHT SEAFOOD, POULTRY, AND MEAT	THE WRONG SEAFOOD, POULTRY, AND MEAT
Fish: All varieties are healthy (with the exception of the large, carnivorous fish), but oily varieties are exceptional. Try salmon, tuna, herring, small mackerel, and lake trout. **Shellfish:** All varieties of shellfish are permissible. **Poultry:** skinless chicken or turkey. Ground turkey breast. **Beef:** lean cuts only. Round steak, cubed steak, London broil, filets, or flank steak. Lean veal is permissible. **Pork:** pork tenderloin or loin chops. Canadian bacon. Prepackaged ham. **Wild Game:** dove, quail, venison, and skinless duck.	**Carnivorous Fish:** swordfish, marlin, shark, tilefish, and king mackerel (high in environmental contaminants). **Processed Meats:** hot dogs, sausages, cold cuts, and regular bacon. **Fatty Cuts** of beef, pork, and lamb, especially ground beef/hamburgers.

The Dairy Section

Ground Rule:

Minimize saturated fat. Choose organic varieties of milk and yogurt.

THE RIGHT DAIRY PRODUCTS	THE WRONG DAIRY PRODUCTS
Milk: skim or 1%. Organic is best. **Soy Milk:** organic, calcium-fortified plain (Silk Enhanced is my top pick). **Yogurt:** Buy low-fat. Plain yogurt has the least amount of sugar. (Stonyfield Farms brand is my top pick.) **Cheese:** part-skim mozzarella and farmer's cheese. Low-fat cottage cheese and low-fat ricotta cheese. Highly flavored cheeses, such as parmesan and feta, are acceptable, as a little goes a long way. Reduced-fat (2% milk) Swiss and cheddar cheeses are also permissible. **Healthy Margarines:** trans fat-free margarine only. (It will be clearly stated on the label.) Look for brand names like Fleishman's Olive Oil Spread, Squeeze Parkay, Brummel and Brown, Smart Balance, Take Control, or Benecol. If available, Smart Balance Plus should be your first choice as it is fortified with omega-3 fats. **Soy Products:** soy cheese, soy hot dogs, tofu, tempeh, etc. are frequently found in the dairy section. **Eggs:** Omega-3 fortified eggs are best. Nature's Design or Eggland's Best are two common brands.	**Whole Fat Dairy:** whole milk, cream, full-fat cheeses, and ice cream. **Fat-Free Fruit Yogurt** **Whipped and Stick Butter** **Stick Margarines and Other Margarines with Trans Fat**

Cereals

Ground Rules:

Only buy 100 percent whole grain and make sure it does not contain hydrogenated oils. Look for cereals with 5 or more grams of fiber per serving and minimal amounts of sugar (10 grams or less per serving). Note: the Right Cereals are listed by brand name.

THE RIGHT CEREALS	THE WRONG CEREALS
Post 100% Bran, Bran Flakes	All junk cereals that break the ground rules
Kashi Seven in the Morning, GoLean, Good Friends, Heart to Heart	
Nature's Path Organic Optimum	
Grape Nuts	
All Bran	
Uncle Sam Cereal	
Kellogg's Complete Wheat Bran Flakes, Complete Oat Bran Flakes, All-Bran, All-Bran Extra Fiber, All-Bran Bran Buds	
Special K Low Carb Lifestyle	
Total Protein	
Wheat Chex, Multi-Bran Chex	
Quaker Oat Squares, Quaker Oat Bran	
Health Valley Golden Flax	
Oatmeal: Old Fashioned (slow-cooking) Oatmeal and steel cut oats are better than the instant varieties, as they have a lower GI. (John McCann's Steel Cut Irish Oats are my top pick.)	

Canned Goods

Ground Rules:

Generally, canned fruits and vegetables are inferior to fresh or frozen counterparts, but some are perfectly fine.

THE RIGHT CANNED GOODS	THE WRONG CANNED GOODS
Acceptable Canned Vegetables: olives, capers, water chestnuts, roasted red peppers, any form of tomato product, artichokes. **Canned Beans:** any variety is acceptable with the exception of fava beans. Keep in mind that the glycemic index of canned beans is higher than their dried counterparts. **Superstar Canned Seafood:** Alaskan salmon (Red Sockeye has most flavor). **Acceptable Canned Seafood:** tuna, crab, shrimp, oysters, and sardines packed in water. (White Albacore tuna has the most omega 3, but is also highest in methyl mercury. Chunk light tuna has the least methyl mercury.)	Canned vegetables that are not on the "right" list **Canned Fruits:** They are all usually packed in sugar.

Frozen Foods

Ground Rules:

Foods that are permissible on the 10 Step Diet are also fine when bought frozen. The two things to consider in the frozen food section are: Are the foods packed in sugar, and would they be allowed if they weren't frozen?

THE RIGHT FROZEN FOODS	THE WRONG FROZEN FOODS
Frozen Vegetables: any permissible vegetable.	Frozen vegetables with added butter, cream, or sauces
Frozen Fruits: any permissible fruits. Frozen berries are just as nutritious as fresh berries, and they are far more economical.	Frozen fruits packed in sugar Breaded/ fried or processed frozen foods
Frozen Skinless Poultry: chicken tenderloins are especially convenient.	
Frozen Seafood: any permissible variety.	
Frozen Whole Grain Waffles: Kashi, Go Lean.	

Nuts and Seeds

Ground Rules:

Go for variety, unless you only like one or two types. Peanuts (legumes, not nuts) are also acceptable.

THE RIGHT NUTS AND SEEDS	THE WRONG NUTS AND SEEDS
Superstar Nuts: almonds, pecans, walnuts, cashews, hazelnuts, Brazil nuts, pistachios, macadamias, pine nuts. **Superstar Seeds:** pumpkin, sunflower, flax, and sesame seeds. **Mixed Nuts:** those without peanuts are best. Wholesale grocers, like Costco, generally have large containers of mixed nuts at a very reasonable price.	**Nuts/Seeds Prepared with Hydrogenated, Partially Hydrogenated, or Other Forbidden Oils.** Check the ingredients on all packaged nuts! **Honey Roasted and Other Varieties Prepared with Sugar**

Oils

Ground Rules:

Buy the monounsaturated oils, and avoid the polyunsaturated oils (corn, safflower, sunflower, soybean) and shortening.

THE RIGHT OILS	THE WRONG OILS
Olive Oil: Extra virgin is the healthiest. **Canola Oil:** If available, "expeller pressed" is the healthiest. **Nut and Seed Oils:** walnut oil, sesame oil, etc. **Cooking Sprays:** canola/olive oil-based cooking sprays, like Pam.	**Corn Oil** **Safflower Oil** **Sunflower Oil** **Soybean Oil (generally referred to as Vegetable Oil)** **Vegetable Shortening (Crisco)**

Rice and Other Grain Dishes

Ground Rules:

Buy whole grain products, rather than refined grain products.

THE RIGHT RICE AND GRAINS	THE WRONG RICE AND GRAINS
Rice: Brown (brown Basmati is best) and authentic wild rice. If you don't like these, then white Basmati, or converted white rice, is your next best choice. **Other Acceptable Grains:** barley, wheat berries, whole wheat bulgur, whole wheat couscous, whole rye, and whole oats.	**White rice and other refined grain dishes**

Pasta

Ground Rules:
Look for whole grain or protein enriched.

THE RIGHT PASTA	THE WRONG PASTA
Whole Wheat Pasta	Traditional Pasta
Protein-Enriched Egg Noodles	Semolina Pasta
	Gluten-Free Pasta

Beans and Legumes

Ground Rules:

Pick any bean you like, except fava beans, which have a very high GI. Remember that dried beans have a lower GI and less sodium than canned beans.

THE RIGHT BEANS AND LEGUMES	THE WRONG BEANS AND LEGUMES
Superstars: lentils, navy beans, kidney beans, split peas, black beans, soybeans, butter beans, and chickpeas (garbanzo beans). **Other Acceptable Beans:** lima, calico, black-eyed peas, pinto beans, cannelloni beans, crowder peas, field peas, red beans, etc.	**Fava Beans**

Baking Products

Ground Rules:

Avoid forbidden ingredients.

THE RIGHT BAKING PRODUCTS	THE WRONG BAKING PRODUCTS
Whole Grain Flours	Refined Flours
Pure Cocoa	
Unsweetened, Bittersweet or Semi-Sweet Dark Chocolate (75% or higher cocoa content is best.)	

Prepared Snack Foods

Ground Rules:

Avoid trans fats (hydrogenated oils), saturated fats (palm, coconut oil), and refined grains like "wheat flour."

THE RIGHT SNACK FOODS	THE WRONG SNACK FOODS
100% Whole Grain Crackers: Wasa, AK MAK, Kashi TLC, etc.	Pretzels, Potato Chips, Corn Chips, Puffed Corn, Popcorn
Pork, Beef, or Turkey Jerky	Crackers made with enriched white flour and/or trans fats (partially hydrogenated oils)
Whole Grain Tortilla Chips: Garden of Eden, Eat Smart, or R.W. Garcia's. (R.W. Garcia's low-carb tortilla chips with flax are my top pick.)	Anything that contains palm or coconut oils (saturated fats)
Roasted Soy Nuts	

Deli/ Bakery

Ground Rules:
Look for lean and fresh deli meats. When buying breads, avoid hydrogenated oils, and only purchase 100 percent whole grain.

THE RIGHT DELI/BAKERY FOODS	THE WRONG DELI/BAKERY FOODS
Fresh Luncheon Meats: turkey, ham, chicken. *Lean* roast beef and pastrami are also acceptable. **Reduced-Fat or 2% Milk Cheeses** **Breads:** Fresh baked 100% whole grain and sourdough are the best. **Permissible Prepackaged Breads:** · Whole grain rye/pumpernickel · Whole grain wraps · Whole grain tortillas · Whole wheat pita bread · Authentic sourdough · Ezekiel Sprouted Grain Bread · Nature's Own 100% Whole Wheat · Cobblestone Mill 100% Whole Grain · Pepperidge Farm Sourdough Wheat · Arnold Melba Thin Rye · Arnold 100% Whole Wheat · Brownberry Natural Health Nut · Arnold Carb Counting 100% Whole Wheat · Thomas' Carb Counting 100% Whole Wheat Bagels **Granola:** homemade only. (Many grocery store bakeries carry this.)	**All Refined Flour Products** **Fatty, Processed Cold Cuts:** bologna, salami, etc.

Nut Butters and Fruit Spreads

Ground Rules:
Avoid hydrogenated oil and added sugar. No high fructose corn syrup.

THE RIGHT NUT BUTTERS AND FRUIT SPREADS	THE WRONG NUT BUTTERS AND FRUIT SPREADS
Peanut Butter: organic or natural brands	**Hydrogenated Oil and Added Sugar:** often found in peanut butter
Almond Butter	
Fruit Spreads: 100% spreadable fruit. (Berry spreads are the best.)	**Jelly, Jams, Marmalade, and Preserves**

Beverages

Ground Rules:
No soda, fruit juice, or sugar-fortified beverages.

THE RIGHT BEVERAGES	THE WRONG BEVERAGES
Bottled Water	All Sodas
Coffee	All Diet Sodas
Loose-leaf Tea: Green tea and black tea are the most healthful.	All Sugar-Fortified Sports Drinks
Vegetable Juice: 100% vegetable juices such as V8, tomato juice.	Fruit Juice Store-Bought Fruit Smoothies
Wine: Red wine is preferable to white wine or rose.	
Beer: low-carbohydrate beer, such as Michelob Ultra, Miller Lite, Rock Green Light, and other light beers.	

Condiments

Ground Rules:
Use these to spike the flavor in foods, and in the case of the acidic varieties, to slow down digestion.

Tip: Have you ever noticed that you feel especially pleasant inside after eating something really hot, like spicy mustard or salsa? When we eat super spicy foods, the pain receptors in our mouths are activated, which leads to the release of endorphins (our bodies' natural morphine) within the brain. When you want a mental lift, go for something hot!

THE RIGHT CONDIMENTS	THE WRONG CONDIMENTS
Lemon or Lime Juice	Full-Fat Mayonnaise
All Vinegars	Regular Ketchup
Tabasco Products	
Hot Sauces	
Mustards	
Herbs and Spices	
Heinz Low-Carb Ketchup	
Light Mayonnaise	
Steak Sauce	
Worcestershire Sauce	
Horseradish	
Capers	
Hot Peppers	
Dill Pickles	
Prepared Guacamole	
Prepared Hummus (and Other Bean Dips)	
Prepared Fresh Salsa	
Teriyaki/Soy Sauce	
Tahini	
Prepared Pesto	
Prepared Tapenade	

Salad Dressing

Ground Rules:

Use a healthy oil base like olive oil or canola oil. If you crave a full-fat salad dressing like blue cheese, mix one part blue cheese to three parts olive oil and vinegar. This way you can get wonderful flavor without all the unhealthy fat.

THE RIGHT SALAD DRESSING	THE WRONG SALAD DRESSING
Homemade Dressing: Use extra virgin olive oil and vinegar or lemon juice. (See Chef Kevin's recipes.) **Annie's Naturals Brands:** Generally, this brand has a healthy oil base. **Vinaigrettes:** Bottled olive oil or canola oil vinaigrettes are best; remember that a little goes a long way. **Reduced-Fat or Light Dressings:** Use as alternatives if you don't like the above.	**Full-Fat (Thicker) Varieties:** ranch, bleu cheese, Thousand Island, etc. A little bit *does not* go a long way, and they frequently have an unhealthy oil base. **Fat-Free Dressings:** They usually contain a lot of sugar.

HOW TO EAT AT HOME

When dieting, you will always have healthier options and quicker results if you prepare most of your meals at home. This chapter includes tips for food preparation that will make implementing the 10-Step Diet easy.

Fruit

- If you buy non-organic fruits, be sure to wash them thoroughly to remove residual fungicides and pesticides. It is best to swirl fruit in diluted soapy water for thirty seconds and rinse thoroughly. If that is impossible, run the fruit under *warm* water.
- Remember that you can find both frozen and fresh, ready-to-eat fruit at most grocery stores. Keep bags of frozen berries in your freezer. Wholesale grocers like Costco and Sam's sell large bags with a convenient zippered opening for a great price.
- Always have one serving of fruit at breakfast and another for a snack. Don't forget to have some healthy protein along with it.

- Berry-based fruit smoothies with soy milk, skim milk, or plain yogurt are delicious and nutritious. Add a hard-boiled omega-3 egg, wheat germ, or flaxseed to enhance it with some healthy omega-3 fats and other beneficial nutrients.

Vegetables

- If you buy non-organic vegetables, make sure you wash or rinse them the same as you do your fruits. (See above.)
- Add vegetables to every dish possible to bulk it up and improve its nutritional value. (For example, I always add fresh garlic, onions, peppers, and carrots to my ground turkey breast spaghetti sauce.)
- One of the most delicious, convenient, and effective ways to ensure that you get the necessary five servings of vegetables a day is to prepare plenty of salads. Use as many vegetables in your salads as possible. Ready-to-use bagged salad greens are super convenient.
- Fresh garlic and onions are great flavor enhancers and contain potent phytochemicals; use them daily in your cooking. Freshly peeled garlic, usually found in the produce section, is a great time saver.
- The healthiest way to cook vegetables is to steam, stir steam, bake, or roast them. Boiling vegetables or cooking them in a microwave will reduce their nutritional value.
- Any type of non-starchy roasted vegetable is delicious. Remember that when you roast vegetables, they dramatically shrink in size; because of this, it is quite simple to get several servings in one sitting. When I roast broccoli for my family (four children and two adults) I use three bundles; when I steam it, one bundle is usually enough.
- Roasting is a fantastic way to use week-old produce that you might not otherwise eat.
- Soups and stews provide a great vehicle for getting more

vegetables into your diet. In the colder months, make some soup each Sunday night. (In the warmer months, try gazpacho.) No matter what the recipe calls for, put all your leftover vegetables in the pot. This way, your vegetable drawer will always be cleaned out for Monday's grocery shopping.

· Having a pre-dinner appetizer of fresh, crunchy vegetable sticks dipped in mustard, oil and vinegar, or hummus is a great habit to develop.

· Enhance the flavor of your vegetables with some trans fat-free margarine, olive oil, lemon juice, vinegar, or Chef Kevin's seasoned salt.

· Pre-cut, bagged vegetables are a great time saver.

· Salad greens, cucumbers, radishes, garlic, and onions are most nutritious when served raw (although garlic and onions retain plenty of their nutritional value even when cooked).

· Serve cruciferous vegetables and fresh spinach either raw or lightly cooked to get the most nutritional benefit.

· Tomatoes, beans, peas, and mushrooms are healthiest when cooked.

· Celery, chives, scallions, asparagus, peppers, and squash are equally nutritious either cooked or raw.

· Habitually season foods with fresh herbs and spices as they offer extremely potent concentrations of powerful phyto-chemicals.

Meats

· Minimize your intake of red meat (especially beef) that has been grilled, broiled, or fried. A known class of carcinogens (heterocyclic amines) can form in the protein fibers of red meat when heated at high temperatures.

· Minimize frying; if you must fry your meats, use canola oil.

· Roasting, pan sautéing, and stewing are the healthiest ways to prepare red meats.

- If eating turkey bacon or center-cut bacon, make sure to cook it in the microwave on a paper towel, rather than in a frying pan. This technique minimizes the saturated fat content.

Omega-3 fortified eggs

- Eggs are healthiest if boiled or poached; however, they are still great for you when prepared other ways.
- Keep a carton of boiled eggs in the refrigerator at all times for a great, grab-and-go protein source.

Soy milk

- Organic calcium fortified soy milk is nutritionally superior to cow's milk. You may not like it by the glass, but you should try it with your whole grain cereal and in your cooking.
- Soy milk is delicious in smoothies.

Oils

- Store all of your oils in the refrigerator (with the exception of olive oil which will harden if you do). When exposed to heat and air, oils will oxidize (become rancid). Oxidized oils are the most potent food source of free radicals (toxic molecules) that we know of. **If an oil or other fatty food (such as peanut butter) smells rancid—throw it out!**
- For this same reason, buy small quantities of oils, and use them quickly. (In other words, it is a bad idea to bring that 5-gallon jug of olive oil home from your Italian vacation and keep it next to your stove six years thereafter.)
- Use olive oil at room temperature or in low heat food preparation.

- In hot food preparation (baking, frying, etc.) it is best to use the more heat-tolerant canola oil.
- If you get into the habit of making your own salad dressings, you will find store-bought varieties inferior in both flavor and taste. It takes no time at all to prepare your own fresh olive oil/canola oil based dressing.

Seafood

- Minimize frying; if you must fry your fish, use canola oil.
- Poached, baked, broiled, pan seared, and sautéed are the best ways to prepare seafood.
- Take advantage of two superstar sources of omega 3s that are always available and convenient: canned Alaskan salmon and sardines.
- Avoid large carnivorous fish (shark, marlin, king mackerel, swordfish, and tilefish) due to pollutants like PCBs, dioxins, and methyl mercury they may contain.
- Although an excellent source of omega 3, fresh tuna should be limited to one serving or less a week because of its moderately high level of methyl mercury. Canned white Albacore tuna should be limited, too.
- Unfortunately, farm raised salmon's fatty-acid profile is not as healthy as its wild counterpart. Additionally, it may have unhealthy concentrations of environmental contaminants (PCBs and dioxins). Choose wild salmon whenever possible.

Nuts/Seeds

- Roast your own. This is the healthiest, tastiest, and most economical way to eat nuts. Simply buy bulk raw nuts/seeds (almonds, pumpkin seeds, walnuts, pecans, etc.), spread them in a single layer on a baking sheet, spray with a thin layer of canola oil, salt as desired, then bake at 350 degrees until the nuts turn golden or slightly brown (about five minutes).

· Store bulk nuts in the freezer to minimize oxidation of their healthy oils.

· Store prepared nuts in the refrigerator.

· To lower the sodium content of store bought salted nuts, dump nuts in a colander, shake vigorously over the sink for a minute or two, and place back in the jar. This removes excess salt.

· Of course, nuts and seeds can also be eaten raw.

Pasta

· Cook *al dente* (slightly undercooked and chewier) to reduce the glycemic index.

· Look for whole-grain pasta or protein-enriched egg noodles.

Beverages

· Drink clean, pure water. Investigate your water source; should you have any doubts about its purity, invest in a home water purification system.

· Keep a bottle of water with you at all times and habitually sip from it over the course of the day.

· Freshly brewed/steeped tea, green or black, is full of anti-aging, immune-boosting antioxidants; drink it regularly. To maximize tea's health benefits, steep it for at least two minutes before you drink it, and squeeze the tea bag at the end of steeping to "wring out" all of the valuable phyto-chemicals.

· The antioxidant power in red wines rivals that found in freshly brewed tea. The red wines with the highest concentration of antioxidant flavonoids include cabernets, merlots, syrahs/shirazes, and zinfandels.

· Remember, a three-quarter cup of V8 or tomato juice counts as a serving of vegetables. This is an easy way to get another vegetable serving into your diet.

Bread

· To reduce its glycemic index, always have your whole grain or sourdough bread with some protein or a healthy fat such as olive oil or a slice of avocado.
· Stop serving bread as a routine accompaniment with your meals.
· Freshly baked sourdough or whole grain breads are available in the bakery sections of most grocery stores, and they taste far superior to pre-packaged breads.

Condiments/Flavor Enhancers

· Use approved condiments freely.
· Lemons, limes, vinegar or vinegar-based sauces, and dressings are excellent for lowering the glycemic index of carbohydrates.
· If a recipe calls for mayonnaise, use half mayo and half plain yogurt; no one will ever know the difference.
· Learn to use yogurt cheese as a substitute for mayonnaise or cream cheese. (See how to make yogurt cheese in Step 5.)

Herbs and spices are a valuable weapon in your weight loss arsenal. Although typically eaten in small amounts, herbs and spices provide flavorful intrigue to most any dish and are helpful in reducing the need for salt and fatty condiments (margarine, etc.) sometimes required in food preparation. What's more, they are teeming with a seemingly endless list of beneficial phytochemicals. According to the USDA nutrient database, parsley has a higher flavonoid concentration than any other food. This refreshing herb also provides vitamin A, potassium, calcium, and vitamin C. Curcumin, the compound that gives turmeric and curry spice their rich, golden-yellow colors, has well documented antioxidant, anti-inflammatory, and anticancer properties. Clover, cinnamon, and bay leaves have recently shown promise in aiding those with type 2 diabetes. Whether you prefer the zing of fresh cilantro or the earthiness of sage, learn to jack up the flavor and healthfulness of your meals with herbs and spices. Fresh herbs offer the most flavor and the highest concentration of phytochemicals, but dried herbs are still plenty powerful.

Soy

· Fermented soy products (tempeh and miso) are especially healthy soy foods.
· Tempeh is extremely versatile and has a fantastic texture. Flavor it with olive oil, black pepper, and balsamic vinegar. It is great in salads or wraps, and if you are like me, you might find tempeh more palatable than tofu.
· Edamame, fresh, whole soybeans, are delicious—try them!
· Roasted soy nuts are a great snack.

Beans and Legumes

· Canned beans are fine, but get into the habit of preparing dried beans in a pressure cooker. Prepared dried beans are far superior in taste, texture, and nutritional value. Most beans can be prepared in twenty minutes or less in the pressure cooker, and there is no need to soak them overnight, a ritual that keeps us from preparing them as often as we should.

· Hummus and other bean dips are great for dipping freshly cut vegetables in or using as a mayo alternative in sandwiches/wraps.

Pressure Cookers: My pressure cooker is my most prized kitchen possession. Today's pressure cookers are completely safe and offer one of the fastest and most nutrient-preserving forms of food preparation available. Almost any meal can be prepared in a fraction of the time it normally takes. If you suffer from time famine like I do, you'll love it! To learn how to become proficient with a pressure cooker, I recommend *Cooking Under Pressure*, by Lorna J. Sass (William Morrow).

DINING OUT ON THE 10 STEP DIET

Who doesn't love dining out? It's fun, easy, and tasty. There is one big problem, though—calories and unhealthy ingredients add up fast when you don't prepare your own food.

While losing weight and dining out are not mutually exclusive, you will run into some considerable challenges. In order stay true to this diet and your wellness goals, you should arm yourself with the following guidelines.

No White Stuff

- Request that bread not be brought to your table, or have it removed as soon as you sit down.
- Ask for salad, beans, or vegetables to replace potatoes, white rice, and pasta sides.
- If your entrée comes with a roll, biscuit, or slices of bread, request that it be held.
- Don't order pasta entrées.

Eat as Many Vegetables as Possible

· Always make salads your meal of choice.
· Seek out restaurants that offer comprehensive salad bars or feature entrée salads. Remember to top your salad with some healthy protein. Opt for olive oil and vinegar as a salad dressing; if that is not available, order low-fat vinaigrettes. Always request that your dressing come on the side so you can control how much goes on your salad. Avoid croutons, full-fat creamy dressings, and full-fat cheese toppings.
· Order bean soups and broth/tomato based vegetable soups.
· If you're not having a salad as your main dish, order a side of vegetables or a small salad.

No Liquid Calories

· Water, unsweetened tea, and coffee are fine.
· A glass of wine, one mixed drink, or one low-carb or light beer is permitted.

Always Include Some Healthy Protein in Your Meal

· Top your salad with some healthy protein—skinless poultry, eggs, nuts, tofu, tempeh, fish, etc.
· If ordering beef or pork, stick to lean cuts only: tenderloin, filets, top round, or top sirloin. No hamburgers, *please*.
· Skinless chicken, seafood, wild game, bean, and egg entrées are all acceptable, as long as they're not fried.

Portion Control (Your *Biggest* Challenge)

· If you know that the restaurant you're dining in serves large portions, request that they be reduced in the kitchen prior to being served.

- Consider an appetizer as your main dish.
- Have your server package half of your meal in a take-home box before you are served, or do it yourself before eating.
- Split an entrée with your dining partner.
- Avoid all-you-can-eat restaurants.
- Stay away from large buffet lines. Studies show that the more variety available to us, the more we eat.

Minimize Unhealthy Fats

- Request that your foods be prepared in canola or olive oil.
- If canola or olive oil is not available, request that all butter, gravy, and sauces be put on the side so you can control your portions.
- Avoid fried foods.
- Stay away from fatty cuts of beef and pork: hamburgers, meat loaf, meat sauces, pork chops, rib eyes, T-bones, New York strips, Porterhouse, ribs, bacon, and sausage.

Your Last Option

If fast food is your only option, don't panic. There are still plenty of choices. Thankfully, many fast food chains are now beginning to recognize the need for healthy alternatives. Still, if you must eat at a fast food restaurant, choose establishments that offer salads and healthy subs or sandwiches. Here's a little guidance when ordering sandwiches, subs, and salads:

- Ask for sourdough or whole grain bread (thinly sliced if available). Whole grain wraps and pita bread are also good.
- Have every vegetable available on your sandwich: lettuce, tomato, pickle, onion, peppers, olives, and so on.
- When available, order veggie sandwiches. If you'd like, request a little lean protein be added.

- If sides come with the sandwich, forget the fries, chips, and pasta salad. Go for coleslaw, bean salad, or fresh fruit.
- If thinly sliced bread is not available, remove one piece before eating.
- Lean turkey, ham, and chicken are acceptable. Lean roast beef is also permissible.
- Use condiments such as mustard, light mayo, oil and vinegar; but stay away from sugar-laden, fat-free sauces.
- When ordering salads, avoid croutons, full-fat cheeses, and fried or breaded chicken.
- Always request vinaigrettes or reduced-fat/light dressings **on the side** so you can control the amount that goes on your salad.

ANSWERS TO DIET QUESTIONS

How much weight will I lose on this diet?

First, keep in mind that there is variability from one person to another on any given weight loss plan depending on an individual's biochemical, genetic, and metabolic makeup. For example, men typically lose weight faster than women, someone who is insulin resistant usually loses weight more slowly than someone who is not, and an individual with a strong family history of obesity may have a harder time than someone without this genetic influence. That said, it is my experience that if you implement all 10 Steps immediately, most people can expect to lose anywhere from 4-6 pounds in the first two weeks. Thereafter, most can expect a 1-2 pound loss weekly. Although not designed to be a "slow" weight loss plan, this is not a fad diet either. Reliable scientific studies now prove that a gradual and steady loss of weight over a protracted period of time increases your odds of maintaining your weight loss; conversely, sudden and rapid weight loss over a short period of time increases the likelihood of gaining back the weight you have lost.

How long will it take before the diet takes effect?

You'll start losing weight right away. You will also experience an immediate and positive change in your energy level and overall sense of well-being.

What if I don't lose weight on this plan?

If you faithfully adhere to all 10 Steps, you will lose weight. If your experience is otherwise, consider writing down and recording what you eat and when you eat it. This will usually reveal where you are going wrong on the dietary portion of this plan. Additionally, be vigilant in your thirty minutes or more of daily exercise, and **wear a pedometer** to ensure you are taking at least ten thousand steps a day.

For some, there may be a metabolic explanation. Some individuals have an under active thyroid gland, a medical condition called hypothyroidism. Hypothyroidism is far from uncommon, and yet it frequently goes undiagnosed. It may explain a person's inability to lose weight, and the condition is especially common among women. Typically, I recommend that all females with weight issues be screened for this condition by having a TSH drawn. In fact, this condition is so common that many physicians, including me, recommend women be screened yearly after the age of forty for hypothyroidism.

What should I do if I don't like fruits or vegetables?

I have found that when you reinforce how good something is for you, it starts to *taste* good. Remind yourself that fruits and vegetables fill you up; they drastically reduce your risk of cancer and heart disease; and finally, lasting weight loss success and lifelong vitality is practically impossible without them.

What's the best way to cook my eggs?

You'll maximize the nutritional benefits of eggs if you eat them either poached or hard-boiled.

Does it matter if I take fish oil capsules or fish oil liquid?

No, as long as you buy a pharmaceutical grade fish oil. Read the packaging to be sure you're not buying a lesser grade. You must see the words "pharmaceutical grade" on the bottle. Pharmaceutical grade fish oil is usually only available at health food stores or organic grocery outlets. Two reputable, national brands that make pharmaceutical grade fish oils are Health from the Sun and Nordic Naturals. You can order their pharmaceutical grade products at nordicnaturals.com (I recommend Ultimate Omega), or health-fromthesun.com (I recommend Ultra Omega 3 Fish Oil + Lipase). Pharmaceutical grade products are optimal because of their quality, potency, and safety.

What's the best way to cook my vegetables?

If you boil your vegetables, nutritious phytochemicals can be damaged and water soluble vitamins, such as vitamins B and C, are leached out. Instead, steam, stir steam, roast, or bake your vegetables. Stir steam by slowly cooking the vegetables in a skillet over low heat in the vegetables' own rendered water. Roast vegetables by spraying them with an olive or canola oil spray, adding a little salt, and roasting at a high temperature (425 degrees) until lightly browned and crispy on the outside.

Can I eat canned vegetables?

The only canned vegetables I recommend for this plan are tomatoes, tomato products, roasted red peppers, and artichokes.

Are frozen vegetables okay to eat?

Fresh, frozen vegetables are absolutely fine.

Are desserts allowed on this diet?

The 10-Step Diet is truly a "diet for life," and I would never expect anyone to go through life without indulging in something sweet. However, if you are serious about weight loss and have a lot of weight to lose, or you are anxious to lose weight as quickly as possible, limit dessert to once a week or less. Once you have reached your weight goals, or if a slower rate of loss is acceptable to you, you can indulge in small portions of healthy sweets more regularly. For some ideas, see Chef Kevin's delicious dessert recipes in Part 4. In the meantime, here are a few healthy sweets:

· Sweeten some plain low-fat yogurt with a little honey or maple syrup, and pour it over fruit; or just enjoy some fruit by itself.
· Try fruit flavored low-fat yogurt when you just have to have something sweet.
· Grab a handful (about 1-1.5 ounces) of semi-sweet chocolate chips or a small piece of high-quality dark chocolate (try Dove Dark, Ghirardelli's semi-sweet baking chips, or another high-quality dark chocolate that is 75 percent or more pure cocoa).
· Hot cocoa (made with cocoa powder and skim or soy milk) is a wonderful treat, especially on those chilly evenings.
· Try sweetened whole grain granola bars; top it with some healthy fat, such as peanut butter or almond butter to lower its glycemic index.

Remember that sweets will be less likely to elevate your blood sugar insulin level if you pair them with some healthy fat or eat them at mealtime—it's not a good idea to have something sweet by itself. Still, it is important to understand that two phys-iological changes will occur when you faithfully follow the 10 Steps. First, your cravings for sweets will dramatically diminish as your insulin levels become lower and more stable; and second, when you reduce your intake of sugar and artificial sweeteners, your taste buds acclimate and become far more sensitive to the taste of sweet. Slightly sweet things become plenty sweet, and sweet things become too sweet.

What if I find it impossible, because of my lifestyle or my love of them, to give up all of the "bad" white stuff?

Do the best you can. Understand and accept that the closer you adhere to the steps, the greater and more rapid your weight loss. If you are unable to completely forgo white rice, white potatoes, and white pasta, then occasionally have smaller amounts as part of a mixed meal that contains protein, fat, fiber, or acid.

If you just can't resist the pull of the "white stuff," here are my specific recommendations for "cheating" on Step 1:

White potatoes

Choose the smaller, new potatoes, and make sure you eat the skin, too. The starch structure of new potatoes is d i f f e r e n t and will not elevate blood glucose quite as much as regular white potatoes. Plus, the skin provides fiber. Prepare them "Greek style" with a little olive oil (fat) and vinegar (acid), and they will be even better.

White rice

Choose converted white rice. It has the lowest glycemic index of all available forms of white rice. Basmati is a good second choice.

Pasta

If you cannot learn to love whole grain pasta, and you just have to have traditional pasta, cook it *al dente*, or to a slightly chewy consistency. This way the pasta will take longer to digest, which reduces its GI.

Even if you can't quit the white carbs entirely, this little cheat sheet should not be abused. Limit yourself to no more than two servings a week of the white carbs for general health purposes. When you do cheat, approach those two servings as a treat and a reward for all your hard work on the other steps.

Why don't you want me to eat corn?

For a vegetable, corn has a relatively high GI, which means it quickly turns to sugar in your system and may cause an unhealthy spike in your blood glucose. Additionally, there are so many other delicious vegetables you can eat on this plan that you needn't miss corn.

You say to minimize tropical fruits like bananas. If I do that, will I get enough potassium?

Absolutely! There's plenty of potassium in the fruits, vegetables, and nuts permitted on this plan.

Is there a difference between farm raised and wild salmon?

About 70 percent of the fresh salmon consumed in this country is farm raised (also known as Atlantic salmon). Although I consider Atlantic salmon to be an important source of valuable omega-3 fats and healthy protein for many Americans, it is inferior in nutritional quality to wild salmon (also called Alaskan salmon). Both have equivalent amounts of omega-3 fat, but farm raised salmon has much more unhealthy saturated fat, a much higher omega 6: omega 3 ratio, and may contain traces of antibiotics and environmental contaminants like PCBs and dioxins. Fresh wild salmon is typically harder to find, but you can usually find it frozen, and you can always find it canned. Wild salmon is always my first choice.

Can I eat canned salmon?

Please do! You'll get the same healthy benefits from canned salmon as fresh salmon. In addition, you can always get wild Alaskan salmon in the can, which is more difficult to find fresh. Red Sockeye has the best flavor.

Does frozen fish have as much nutritional value as fresh?

Yes, there's minimal to no nutritional difference between fresh and frozen fish.

Seven servings of fruits and vegetables a day is a lot. How do you suggest I incorporate them into a typical day?

First, always keep them "top of mind." Build your entire meal around vegetables. Always have one serving of fruit at breakfast and one serving later in the day as part of a meal or a snack. Remember to combine it with some healthy protein when snacking. Have one serving of vegetables at breakfast; try peppers, garlic, onion, tomatoes, avocados, tomato juice, or V8. Routinely have a large salad, with as many vegetables as possible, for lunch or dinner. If you are not going to have a salad at mealtime, always have at least two vegetable servings as side dishes. Make raw veggies part of your daily snack routine.

I love eggs, but am worried about the cholesterol. What do you suggest?

Eggs are an exceptional food; they are low in saturated fat, contain beneficial fats, the highest quality protein available, and several very important essential nutrients, like vitamin E, B-12, and folate. They do contain relatively high amounts of cholesterol, but we now know that saturated fats and trans fat are the real culprits in our cholesterol-elevating diets. A small percentage of individuals with high cholesterol can experience an elevation if they eat too many eggs, but most will not. If you have a cholesterol problem, play it safe; limit your intake to seven eggs a week. If you don't have elevated cholesterol, have as many eggs as you like. Remember, though, that the eggs I recommend are even healthier because they contain omega-3 fats. My anecdotal experience is that these special eggs can actually improve your cholesterol profile. Omega-3 eggs are a healthier choice than egg substitutes, too.

What's better for me as a source of omega 3-flaxseed oil or fish oil?

I recommend fish oil over flax oil as a supplemental source of omega-3 fats because it contains the longer chained omega-3 fatty acids, DHA and EPA, in their preformed states—meaning that they are already in a "ready-to-use" form for your body. Flax oil is a rich source of a shorter chain omega-3 fat, called alpha-linolenic acid (ALA), which has no known specific function in the body other than providing the building blocks for the longer chained omega-3 fats like DHA and EPA. Unfortunately, in humans the conversion of ALA into the longer chained omega 3s is inefficient (generally no higher than 12-14 percent at best).

If I eat tuna, should I worry about methyl mercury?

Fresh tuna and canned white Albacore tuna contain moderately high levels of methyl mercury. I recommend you limit these two varieties of tuna to one serving per week. I would discourage sensitive populations—pregnant women, nursing women, and children under the age of six—from eating fresh tuna or white Albacore tuna more than once a month.

I love peanut butter. Do I have to give it up?

Not at all! Peanut butter in moderation is perfectly acceptable. However, for variety and health benefits, I suggest you try almond butter or other nut butters, too. Nonetheless, when buying peanut butter, check the label and choose those brands that **do not** contain hydrogenated oils or added sugar.

What would you consider to be the top ten healthiest foods?

It is difficult to narrow it down to just ten because we are blessed with so many nutritional superstars. Nonetheless, if I had to choose, here is my top-ten list:

1. Blueberries
2. Wild Alaskan salmon (canned is fine)
3. Almonds
4. Kale
5. Red onions
6. Spinach
7. Oranges
8. Whole oats
9. Broccoli
10. Extra virgin olive oil

Do you recommend dietetic sweeteners?

As a general rule, no—even for those who are trying to lose weight. Although there is no scientific evidence that they have any long-term, negative health consequences, thousands of people have reported side effects from the use of some brands of dietetic sweeteners. Further, there is scant evidence proving dietetic sweeteners help people in their weight loss endeavors.

Keep in mind that the taste of something sweet is sometimes enough to cause your pancreas to release insulin. For those who have carbohydrate sensitivity (insulin resistance), dietetic sweeteners can potentially trigger their pancreases to release insulin into their systems. Additionally, animal studies have shown that the unsatisfied expectation of calories (as in the case of zero calorie dietetic sweeteners) may affect the brain in a way that actually *increases* appetite. A final concern about dietetic sweeteners is their potential to exploit our highly developed sense of taste for sweet things. The popular brands are two to six hundred times sweeter than table sugar. As such, the bar for what tastes sweet gets set very high. I have doubts that a juicy orange or a cup of plump blueberries will satisfy your sweet tooth if you regularly partake in these exquisitely sweet substances.

If you must have something sweeter than what is allowed on this plan, I prefer you use a small amount of the real thing. If you insist on the use of artificial sweeteners, use sucralose (Splenda). Based on my personal research, I am most medically comfortable with this specific brand.

Because insulin resistance syndrome severely compromises my weight loss efforts and my health in general, what are all of the known changes I can make in my diet and lifestyle to overcome it?

All of the following have been shown to reduce, and in many cases, completely alleviate insulin resistance syndrome.
- Establishing and maintaining normal body weight (BMI of 24 or less).
- Engaging in regular exercise—30 minutes or more of moderate aerobic activity, 5 or more days a week.
- Avoiding trans fats.
- Minimizing saturated fat.
- Increasing dietary fiber from whole grains and beans.
- Reducing caloric intake in general.
- Minimizing the highly refined, high glycemic index carbohydrates.
- Increasing omega-3 fats.

Am I missing any nutritional benefits if I eat berries that have been frozen?

Not at all. In fact, in some instances, frozen berries may be more potent than fresh berries. When picking their crop in order to flash freeze it, growers typically wait until berries are at their absolute peak of ripeness. And it's during the last week or so of ripening that many of the most beneficial phytochemicals increase in concentration.

What can I use in place of butter?

Look for margarines with packages that clearly state "contains no trans fat." These are margarines that are more liquid at room temperature and can be found in all grocery stores.

What foods do you think are the absolute worst to eat on this diet, when it comes to elevating blood glucose and insulin levels?

Here is my top ten list of the worst carbohydrate foods. Standard American servings of these foods typically send glucose levels soaring.

1. Pancakes with syrup
2. Baked russet potatoes
3. Regular beer
4. White rice
5. White bagels
6. Macaroni and cheese
7. Pop Tarts
8. Standard American pizza
9. Pretzels
10. Corn Flakes

My all-time pick of the *absolute unhealthiest foods* are *glazed donuts* and fast food *french fries*. Both are loaded with trans fat and are comprised of the worst carbohydrates: refined white flour and sugar for glazed donuts, and white potato starch for french fries. In addition, they contain little or no fiber, no phytochemicals, and few essential nutrients.

Can I include diet soft drinks on this diet?

I strongly discourage you from drinking diet sodas on a regular basis. Regular consumption of diet sodas is an unhealthy habit.

Most contain caffeine, a highly addictive chemical that keeps you coming back for more, and they have no nutritionally redeeming qualities. Valuable minerals in your body, such as calcium, must buffer their acidic makeup. Over time, this may predispose you to osteoporosis. This same acid can also erode your tooth enamel. Finally, extremely carbohydrate-sensitive individuals may release insulin into their bloodstreams in response to the mere taste of something sweet, regardless of its calorie content. If you sip two or three diet sodas a day, you may be continuously priming your bloodstream with that fat-loving hormone, insulin. One of my most successful weight loss clients dropped 12 pounds in two months simply by staying away from diet sodas and other artificially sweetened products.

Please, drink water instead.

Are raw vegetables better for me than cooked ones?

Some vegetables are better for you raw, while others are better for you cooked. Your best bet is to eat some of both.

If I consume a lot of oily fish, do I need to take a fish oil supplement?

According to most experts, if you regularly and consistently consume three healthy servings of oily fish each week, supplements are not necessary. Because most people don't succeed in this regard, I recommend everyone supplement their diets with pharmaceutical grade fish oil as a general rule. To be most cost efficient, on the days you do have a serving of oily fish, you can omit your supplement.

Can I include peanuts as part of my daily handful of nuts and seeds?

Strictly speaking, peanuts are legumes, not nuts. Feel free to eat them, but stay away from beer nuts or candy-coated peanuts.

Why do you want me to eat protein at every meal?

Compared to carbohydrates, the digestion of protein promotes a more prolonged, steady blood glucose level. A stable blood glucose level means less hunger. In addition, protein can slow the rate of stomach emptying, an added plus when you're eating a moderate to high GI carb.

You suggest drinking 100 percent vegetable juice like V8. Doesn't that have a lot of added salt?

In the context of this eating plan, it is not enough to cause you concern.

On your list of suggested fruits, you include dried apricots. Don't dried fruits have a lot of sugar?

With the exception of apricots, all dried fruits have a very high glycemic index and should be avoided by those trying to lose weight. The high fiber content of apricots, however, dramatically slows their digestion, giving them a much lower GI.

If I exercise without changing my diet, will I get any health benefits?

Any amount of exercise you do will change your life. If you've spent your life being sedentary and feel that thirty minutes of aerobic exercise is out of your reach, then walk five or ten minutes and build up to thirty. Aerobic exercise, like walking, is one of the best things you can do for your health. Obviously, if you walk and continue to eat trans fat and high glycemic index carbs, you'll minimize the positive effects of exercise. However, some exercise is absolutely better than none.

If I diet but don't exercise, will I lose weight?

Yes, but at a slower rate, especially if you have insulin resistance.

Can I use mayonnaise?

Sure, but try a light brand. If your recipe calls for mayonnaise, mix half light mayonnaise with half plain low-fat yogurt—no one will be able to tell the difference. Consider the use of yogurt cheese for the healthiest and most weight loss friendly mayo substitute.

I'm not very good at thinking up meals. If I fix a tuna sandwich on whole grain bread for lunch, what else can I include in the meal?

See Chef Kevin's great menu ideas in Part 4.

What's better to use: margarine or butter?

Standard stick margarine is loaded with trans fat and worse than butter. Trans fat-free margarines are a healthier choice than butter, as butter contains lots of unhealthy saturated fat.

What do you think are the most palatable ways to eat soy products?

Most people find roasted soy nuts and edamame (fresh green soybeans) delicious. I also find that most of my clients are successful substituting soy milk for cow's milk in cereal. I recommend that you experiment with all of the available soy products to see which ones you like the best.

What about frozen produce?

Frozen produce is both a healthy and acceptable alternative to fresh produce; however, avoid frozen fruits packed in sugar.

Are there any types of fish that I should not eat?

Unfortunately, the larger, carnivorous fish—shark, marlin, tilefish, king mackerel, and swordfish—can be very high in environmental contaminants like PCBs, methyl mercury, and dioxins. For this reason, I recommend that you avoid them completely.

Why is "extra virgin" olive oil the healthiest oil?

"Extra virgin" means that it has been obtained in the first pressing of the olives. This form of olive oil contains higher levels of a potent antioxidant called squalene and is less likely to contain oxidized fatty acids, which can be toxic.

What is "expeller pressed" canola oil?

"Expeller pressed" means the oil has been extracted from its natural source—in this case, the rape plant—by physical pressure, rather than the use of heat and chemical solvents. Heat and chemical extraction can cause oxidation, which can damage healthy fats. Expeller pressed oils, if available, are the healthiest choice.

What do you think about using meal replacement bars?

Because I prefer people to obtain their nutrients and calories from whole foods, I'm not enthusiastic about meal replacement bars. They definitely qualify as processed foods. However, to have them on occasion is perfectly acceptable.

What about microwaving foods?

I recommend using the microwave only to heat or reheat foods. Cooking foods in this way, especially produce, can reduce their nutritional value. Always use microwave-safe glass or ceramic containers, not plastic, and don't use plastic wraps. Potentially hazardous molecules in plastics can be transferred into microwaved foods.

I keep hearing about a dangerous medical condition called metabolic syndrome. What is it?

Metabolic syndrome is a recently recognized and increasingly common (30percent of U.S. adults have it) medical diagnosis characterized by a constellation of several metabolic risk factors occurring simultaneously in one individual. These metabolic factors include central obesity (excessive fat in the belly), abnormal blood lipids (high triglycerides, low HDL, high cholesterol), high blood pressure, and insulin resistance. If you have metabolic syndrome, your risk of heart attack, stroke, and type 2 diabetes is severely increased. Weight loss, exercise, and a healthy diet (i.e. the 10 Steps) can alleviate the syndrome in most people.

Part 3
Customize the 10 Steps
for Prevention

DISEASE PREVENTION

As you know by now, the 10 Step Diet is not simply about looking great and feeling great, but about *getting* well and *staying* well. Predictably, these ideas go hand in hand.

If you're overweight or obese, you are at risk of developing a life-threatening illness. Years ago, little was known about the correlation between weight and major disease; today, however, the link is clear. Being overweight or obese significantly increases your chances of a host of modern day ills, from heart attacks to type 2 diabetes and even most types of cancer. Just this past year, the Centers for Disease Control released a statement asserting that obesity is fast on the heels of smoking as the number one cause of preventable deaths in this country. As a physician I am horror struck by this ominous reality, especially as most people are still unaware of the dangers of excess body fat. Losing weight can save your life.

What follows is the "extended version" of the 10-Step Diet. Specifically, I have taken the ten most common chronic diseases for which being overweight places you at an increased risk and provided all of the known dietary and lifestyle strategies you can employ to avoid them. This section, therefore, provides the 10 Steps *you* need to take to prevent these conditions or minimize their impact if you already have them. As you will quickly see, there is considerable overlap within the "prevention steps," and the diet itself. Given that this plan was designed with the intentions of maximizing the wellness and vitality of those I personally engage with as a physician and a wellness expert, this is likely far from surprising. If you have been diagnosed with any of the following conditions, or if after reviewing the specific risk factors listed for each disease you find that you are at increased risk of developing any of these illnesses, I urge you to follow the outlined steps in order to ensure your optimum health, and to consult with your physician for a medical evaluation.

Cancer Is a Killer

"Cancer" is a catchall term to describe a group of diseases caused by the uncontrolled growth and spread of abnormal cells. Cancer can be caused by both external (tobacco, chemicals) and internal (hormones, genes) factors. According to the American Cancer Society, 556,500 Americans perished in 2003 from some form of cancer—that's about 1,500 people every single day in our country alone. In the same year, over a million new cancers were reported. Cancer is the second leading cause of death in the United States, exceeded only by heart disease.

Who is at risk? Unfortunately, we all are; however, certain factors can increase the likelihood of developing cancer.

- Advancing age: The chances of virtually all cancers increase as we age.
- Tobacco use: Male smokers are twenty times more at risk of developing lung cancer as nonsmokers, and female smokers are twelve times more at risk than nonsmokers.
- Heredity: 5-10 percent of cancers have a hereditary component. The big ones are colon, breast, prostate, and ovarian cancers.

- Obesity: According to the National Cancer Institute, obesity appears to increase the risk of cancers of the breast, colon, prostate, endometrium (lining of the uterus), cervix, ovary, kidney, and gallbladder.
- Poor diets: Diets low in fruit, vegetables, and fiber, and high in saturated fats, trans fats, red meat, refined carbohydrates, and calories.
- Alcohol abuse
- Physical inactivity

Is cancer preventable? In many cases, absolutely. You can avoid five of the seven previous risk factors by modifying your diet and lifestyle. In addition, getting regular exams and screenings can frequently result in early detection, especially of breast, colon, rectal, cervical, prostate, testis, oral, and skin cancers. Cancers that are detected by routine screenings account for nearly half of all new cancers diagnosed annually.

In an American Institute of Cancer Research report (*Food, Nutrition and the Prevention of Cancer: A Global Perspective*, 1997), it was shown that diet plays a major role in cancer prevention. In fact, in this study, scientists found that 30-40 percent of cancers are directly linked to diet and related factors, such as physical inactivity. Similarly, in a study of nearly one million adults conducted by the American Cancer Society, researchers estimated that more than ninety thousand cancer deaths could be avoided each year if Americans maintained a healthy weight. **If you eat right, stay active, and watch your weight, you can actually decrease your risk of cancer by 30-40 percent.**

1. **Consume as many fruits and vegetables as possible;** aim for seven or more servings a day.

Over two hundred studies have illustrated the anticancer power of fruits and vegetables. Consume the superstar fruits for cancer protection: apples with their skins, berries, pomegranates, avocados, and all whole citrus. Oranges are especially good, as they contain one of the most comprehensive cocktails of cancer-fighting phytochemicals.

Consume the superstar vegetables: all cruciferous vegetables (broccoli, cabbage, brussels sprouts, cauliflower—most potent when eaten raw); allium vegetables, (garlic, onions, leaks, chives, scallions—most potent when chopped); dark leafy greens (spinach, kale, collards, dark green lettuce); carrots, tomatoes, asparagus, and butternut squash.

2. **Avoid overnutrition (also known as "overeating").** Overeating has been associated with an increased cancer risk. Watching your caloric intake is a powerful way to prevent cancer.

3. **Exercise regularly.** There is solid evidence that regular exercise protects against breast, colon, and prostate cancer. As medical science progresses, we can be certain that other cancers will be added to this list.

4. **Limit consumption of red meat (beef, pork, lamb) to two servings or less a week.** Red meat, alas, is not very good for us. When meat is cooked at high temperatures (grilling, barbecuing, frying, broiling) a known class of carcinogens, heterocyclic amines (HCAs) can materialize. Further, meat can be a source of nitrosamines, another kind of carcinogen, which can form in the gastrointestinal tract when cured meats (ham, hot dogs, bologna, salami) are consumed.

In addition, meats are a concentrated source of iron, absorbed into your body whether you need it or not. Studies show a positive relationship between high blood levels of iron and certain cancers. Finally, meats are high on the food chain, where potentially hazardous environmental chemicals, such as hormones, pesticides, and fungicides concentrate.

5.   **Do your carbs right by minimizing your intake of the high glycemic varieties (white flour, white rice, white potatoes, and sugar).** Excessive consumption of high glycemic index carbs can lead to elevated blood insulin levels, which can trigger hormonal changes encouraging cellular growth. Replace high glycemic index carbs with fruits and vegetables, beans (especially soybeans), and whole grains.

6.   **Do your fats right!** Minimize consumption of omega-6 fats (sunflower, safflower, corn, and cottonseed oils), saturated fats, and trans fats. Maximize your intake of omega-3 fats, especially from oily fish (salmon, tuna, mackerel, sardines, lake trout, and herring). Consume monounsaturated oils (canola, olive oil, nuts/seeds, avocados) as your primary fat source, as these foods have potential anticancer properties. Specifically, canola oil is a good source of omega-3 fats; extra virgin olive oil is a potent source of antioxidant polyphenols, including squalene; and nuts and seeds provide you with the cancer protective mineral, selenium.

7.   **Limit alcohol consumption: one drink or less per day for women and two drinks or less per day for men.** Alcohol consumption has been shown to increase the risk of colon, throat, esophageal, uterine, cervical, oral, breast, and liver cancers. In the famous Nurses' Health Study (Harvard), women who had two drinks a day increased their risk of breast cancer by 20-25 percent.

8.   **Minimize exposure to potential environmental carcinogens:** tobacco products, fungicides, pesticides, herbicides, industrial pollutants (PCBs, dioxins, methyl mercury), household cleaning products, excessive food dyes or coloring, and radiation (unnecessary x-rays or nuclear studies).

     Drink pure, clean water, either bottled or from a water purification system. Buy organic produce if you can afford it. If not, thoroughly wash and rinse all produce. (See Part 2: How to Eat at Home on recommended methods.)

9. **Consume lots of tea, turmeric, curry, and ginger.** Maximize your catechin intake (a group of antioxidant phytochemicals) by drinking freshly brewed tea steeped for two minutes. Flavor your food with turmeric, ginger, and curry; all contain potent phytochemicals that show promise in cancer protection.

10. **Take your supplements daily!** A multivitamin, 500-1,000 mg of vitamin C in divided doses, 400 IU of vitamin E, and pharmaceutical grade fish oil. (See the next chapter for additional information on supplements.) Also take 200 mcg of the mineral selenium or eat one to two Brazil nuts as an alternative. (If you have a chronic medical condition or take prescription drugs, consult your physician first.)

Just Quit!

In 2003, more than 180,000 deaths were expected to be caused by tobacco. Smoking is the single most preventable cause of death in our country, and tobacco is one of the most addictive drugs in the world. **All cancers caused by smoking are preventable.**

Tobacco can:

- Damage your lungs (emphysema) and contribute to all forms of respiratory illness.

- Cause cancer of the lung, bladder, mouth, throat, kidney, esophagus, and neck.

- Contribute to premature wrinkling of the skin, impotence, loss of stamina, and energy.

- Cause all forms of cardiovascular disease including heart attack, stroke, high blood pressure, and peripheral vascular disease.

Here is the good news: if you currently smoke, the damaging effects of tobacco on the cardiovascular system are mostly reversible. Please take advantage of this amazing fact and quit.

---

10 STEPS TO PREVENT BREAST CANCER

Are You at Risk?

The American Cancer Society estimates that in 2004, more than 266,000 new cases of breast cancer will be diagnosed in women and 1,300 in men. Those statistics make breast cancer the most frequently diagnosed non-skin cancer in women, as well as the second highest cause of cancer deaths in women. In one year alone, the disease will kill an estimated 40,200 women.

The risk of breast cancer increases with age. Other factors increasing risk include:
- Obesity
- Family history, especially in a first degree relative
- Not having a child before the age of thirty
- Post-menopausal estrogen and progestin use
- Alcohol use
- Long menstrual history (early onset, late cessation)

The American Cancer Society recommends that women over forty have an annual mammogram and clinical exam by a healthcare professional. Changing how you live and what you eat can also protect you from developing breast cancer.

1. **Consume as many fruits and vegetables as possible.** Eat seven or more servings daily. The superstars for breast cancer protection include all cruciferous vegetables (broccoli, cabbage, brussels sprouts, cauliflower); dark leafy greens (collards, kale, spinach); carrots and tomatoes. The superstar fruits include citrus, berries, and cherries. Note: it is best to eat cruciferous vegetables raw or lightly cooked, as some of the phytochemicals believed to offer protection against breast cancer are destroyed by heat.

2. **Limit alcohol consumption to one drink or less a day.** The Harvard Nurses' Health Study, along with several others, has shown consuming more than one alcoholic beverage a day can increase breast cancer risk by as much as 20-25 percent.

3. **Do your carbs right by minimizing your intake of the high glycemic varieties (white flour, white rice, white potatoes, and sugar).** Excessive consumption of high glycemic index carbs can lead to elevated blood insulin levels, which can trigger hormonal changes encouraging cellular growth. Replace high glycemic index carbs with fruits and vegetables, beans, soy products, and whole grains.

4. **Exercise regularly the rest of your life.** Multiple studies have shown that regular exercise is a powerful strategy to fight breast cancer.

5. **Do your fats right!** Minimize consumption of omega-6 fats (sunflower, safflower, corn, and cottonseed oils), saturated fats, and trans fats. Maximize your intake of omega-3 fats, especially from oily fish (salmon, tuna, mackerel, sardines, lake trout, and herring). Consume monounsaturated oils (canola, olive oil, nuts/seeds, avocados) as your primary fat

source, as these foods have potential anticancer properties. Specifically, canola oil is a good source of omega-3 fats; extra virgin olive oil is a potent source of antioxidant polyphenols, including squalene; and nuts and seeds provide you with the cancer protective mineral, selenium.

6. **Eat your beans.** Beans have been associated with reduced breast cancer risk. They are an excellent source of folic acid and lignans, both compounds with potent anticancer features.

7. **Consume whole food soy products regularly, such as tofu, tempeh, edamame, roasted soy nuts, soy milk, and miso.** Only consume organic, non-GMO (genetically modified) soy. Epidemiologic studies have shown a positive association between soy consumption and reduced breast cancer risk. I recommend women at risk for breast cancer consume several servings of soy foods a week.

8. **Minimize exposure to pharmacologic estrogens and xeno-estrogens.** Do not take prescription estrogens unless medically indicated. Lifetime exposure to estrogen plays a fundamental role in the development of breast cancer. Also avoid estrogen-like compounds found in environmental pollutants, such as pesticides and industrial chemicals. Buy organic produce if you can afford it; otherwise, thoroughly wash all non-organic produce (see Part 2: How to Eat at Home). Minimize exposure to residual hormones found in non-organic dairy products, meat, and poultry.

9. **Take your supplements daily.** A multivitamin, 500-1,000 mg of vitamin C in divided doses, 400 IU of vitamin E, and pharmaceutical grade fish oil. Also take 200 mcg of the mineral selenium or eat one to two Brazil nuts as an alternative. (See the next chapter for additional information on supplements.) If you have a chronic medical condition or take prescription drugs, consult your physician first.

10. **Maintain a positive mental outlook.** Engage in self-nurturing behaviors regularly. Develop rich, warm, and mutually beneficial relationships with family and friends. The mind-body associations with breast cancer are significant.

Be Proactive!

1. Give yourself a monthly breast self-examination.

2. Get a yearly examination by a healthcare professional.

3. Have a mammogram yearly over the age of forty or as directed by your doctor.

---

10 STEPS TO PREVENT PROSTATE CANCER

Men at Risk

Prostate cancer is the second leading cause of cancer deaths in men. Although overall death rates have been on the decline since the early 1990s, African-American males are still twice as likely to die from prostate cancer as Caucasian males. Yearly prostate specific antigen (PSA) testing, along with a digital rectal exam, is recommended for all men over fifty and for men at high risk, including black males and those with a positive family history, at the age of forty.

Doctors at the University of California, Los Angeles, report that prostate cancer is ten times more common in the United States than in Japan. Preliminary findings suggest the difference may be diet. When Japanese men move to the United States and eat a high-fat American diet their risk of prostate cancer increases. Aside from saturated fat content, one of the biggest differences found in American and Japanese diets is the predominance of soy foods in native Japanese diets. Many experts believe soy may offer protection against prostate cancer.

Nutrition also came into play in a study reported in the *Journal of the National Cancer Institute* (November 6, 2002, Volume 94 (21)) that showed a diet rich in garlic, shallots, and onions (the allium food group) may cut the risk of prostate cancer in half. This study, conducted on male residents of Shanghai, showed that those who ate more than a third of an ounce from the allium food group daily were 50 percent less likely to have prostate cancer.

Risk factors for prostate cancer include:
· Advancing age
· African American race
· Family history in a first degree relative
· Some studies indicate that dietary fat may also be a factor

1. **Consume ten or more tomato products a week.** A 1995 Harvard Medical School study that surveyed 48,000 male health professionals revealed that men who consumed ten or more tomato products a week (tomato sauce, juice, ketchup, salsa, or tomatoes themselves) reduced their risk of life-threatening prostate cancer by 50 percent (*Journal of the National Cancer Institute*, December 6, 1995, Volume 87 (23)). It is believed that the powerful antioxidant, lycopene, a phytochemical found in high concentrations in tomatoes, was the magic ingredient in this healthy recipe. Cooked tomato products (sauce, paste) served with a little oil are the very best sources of lycopene.

2. **Minimize your intake of animal products high in saturated fat: fatty cuts of beef, pork, and lamb.** Diets high in saturated animal fats have been associated with an increased risk of prostate cancer.

3. **Do not overeat.** A study published in the 2003 issue of *Urology* (Volume 61), which included 444 middle-aged and senior men, found that those with the highest caloric intakes

were four times more likely to develop prostate cancer, compared to those who consumed the fewest calories.

4. **Consume whole food soy products regularly, such as soy milk, tofu, tempeh, miso, edamame, and roasted soy nuts.** Epidemiological and laboratory studies have shown soy foods to be protective against prostate cancer. It is believed that this is related to a class of phytochemicals called isoflavones, abundant in soy foods. The Seventh Day Adventist study, which included 12,395 California males, showed that those who frequently consumed soy milk (more than once a day) had a 70 percent reduced risk of prostate cancer (*Cancer Causes & Control*, December 1998, Volume 9 (6)).

5. **Eat as many fruits and vegetables as possible for general anti-cancer protection.** Aim for seven or more servings a day. The superstar vegetables for prostate cancer prevention include: asparagus, tomatoes, winter squash, sweet potatoes, and anything in the allium family (garlic, onions, scallions, chives, leeks). The superstar fruits for prostate cancer protection include red grapefruit, guava, and watermelon.

6. **Exercise regularly.** Studies show that men who exercise regularly have lower rates of prostate cancer.

7. **Do your carbs right by minimizing your intake of the high glycemic varieties (white flour, white rice, white potatoes, and sugar).** High glycemic index carbohydrates can lead to elevated blood insulin levels, which, in turn, can increase levels of hormones that may promote cancerous growth in the prostate. Choose fruit, vegetables, beans, and whole grains instead.

8. **Do your fats right!** Minimize consumption of omega-6 fats (sunflower, safflower, corn, and cottonseed oils), saturated fats, and trans fats. Maximize your intake of omega-3 fats, especially from oily fish (salmon, tuna, mackerel, sardines, lake trout, and herring). Consume monounsaturated oils

(canola, olive oil, nuts/seeds, avocados) as your primary fat source, as these foods have potential anti-cancer properties. Specifically, canola oil is a good source of omega-3 fats; extra virgin olive oil is a potent source of antioxidant polyphenols, including squalene; and nuts and seeds provide you with the cancer protective mineral, selenium.

9. **Minimize consumption of animal products high in calcium: cheese and cow's milk.** Drink soy milk instead. Excessive dietary calcium from animal sources has been associated with an elevated prostate cancer risk.

10. **Take your supplements and low dose aspirin daily.** A multivitamin, 500-1,000 mg of vitamin C in divided doses, 400 IU of vitamin E, pharmaceutical grade fish oil, and 200 mcg of the mineral selenium, or eat one to two Brazil nuts as an alternative. (See the next chapter for additional information on supplements.) If you have a chronic medical condition or take prescription drugs, consult your physician first. Take 81 mg of aspirin daily. A recent report (*British Journal of Cancer*, January 12, 2004, Volume 90 (1)) analyzed data from twelve studies and found that regular use of aspirin was associated with a 30 percent reduction in the risk of advanced prostate cancer and 10 percent reduction in total prostate cancer risk. (Consult with your physician before taking aspirin regularly.)

10 STEPS TO PREVENT AND MINIMIZE TYPE 2 DIABETES

An American Epidemic

Diabetes occurs when your body does not produce or properly use insulin, the hormone needed to allow glucose and other fuels to enter your cells. Currently more than 17 million Americans have diabetes, or approximately 6.2 percent of the population. Additionally, it was recently reported that an astounding 40 percent of Americans above the age of forty are pre-diabetic. Obesity and a sedentary lifestyle are the leading risk factors for developing type 2 diabetes, and nearly 85 percent of newly diagnosed type 2 diabetics are overweight. A positive family history and consumption of trans fats are the other risk factors for this condition.

Complications of diabetes include:
- · Kidney disease
- · Blindness
- · Heart attack
- · Stroke
- · Nerve damage
- · Peripheral vascular disease (loss of limbs, impotence, etc.)

According to the American Diabetic Association, two out of three diabetics die from heart disease or stroke. Diabetes frequently goes undiagnosed in the early stages because minimal symptoms are present. Symptoms of well-developed type 2 diabetes include: frequent urination, excessive thirst, extreme hunger, unusual weight loss, increased fatigue, irritability, and blurry vision. Type 2 diabetes can be prevented and in some cases reversed; all you have to do is make changes in the way you live and eat. A landmark multi-center study published in the *New England Journal of Medicine* (February 7, 2002, Volume 346 (6)) found that individuals who lost a modest 7 percent of their body weight and engaged in thirty minutes of moderate, aerobic activity (walking) five days a week reduced their risk of type 2 diabetes by 58 percent. Experts believe that 90 percent of all cases of type 2 diabetes cases can be prevented through dietary modifications, weight loss, and an increased activity level.

1. **Maintain an optimal weight.** To avoid type 2 diabetes, strive to maintain an optimal weight. This is the most powerful strategy to decrease your risk of developing type 2 diabetes, or if you already have it, to minimize its impact.

2. **Exercise regularly for the rest of your life.** This is the second most powerful strategy to avoid or control type 2 diabetes. Your optimal regimen should include thirty minutes or more of aerobic activity five or more days a week. Lifting weights has also been shown to be beneficial.

3. **Strictly avoid or minimize the high glycemic white carbohydrates: white flour, white rice, sugar, and white potatoes.** Consumption of white carbs leads to sudden elevations in blood glucose and insulin levels, which promotes weight gain and damages your cardiovascular system. When consumed over time, white carbohydrates encourage insulin resistance and may lead directly to the development of type 2 diabetes in susceptible individuals.

4. **Do your fats right!** Minimize saturated and strictly avoid trans fats. Saturated and trans fat contribute to heart disease and insulin resistance, the underlying metabolic problem in type 2 diabetes. Stay healthy by consuming the majority of your fats from the monounsaturated oils (extra virgin olive oil, canola oil, nuts, seeds, and avocados) and foods containing omega-3 fats (salmon, tuna, herring, mackerel, sardines, walnuts, soy, flax seed, wheat germ, and omega-3 eggs).

5. **Consume your carbohydrates from the low to moderate glycemic index sources: vegetables, beans and legumes, fruit, and whole grains.** Eat as many vegetables as possible, with the goal of at least five servings a day. All vegetables are great with the exception of starchy varieties, such as corn, potatoes, parsnips, and rutabagas. Vegetable superstars, for the prevention of type 2 diabetes, include: onions, broccoli, okra, brussels sprouts, dark leafy greens, tomatoes, and red and yellow peppers.

   Limit fruit to two servings daily, as they contain natural sugars which can elevate blood glucose and insulin levels. Avoid the sweeter, tropical fruits: bananas, mangos, pineapples, and papayas. The best fruits are berries (all varieties), cherries, apples, whole citrus, pears, plums, red grapes, apricots (dried or fresh), and peaches.

   Consume your grain products (cereals and breads) strictly from whole grain sources. The best whole grains for those concerned with type 2 diabetes are barley, rye, and oats.

   Strive to have one serving of beans or legumes a day. Although there are more than twenty-four varieties of beans available, choose those with the lowest glycemic index: soybeans, lentils, kidney beans, pinto beans, navy beans, chickpeas, black beans, and butter beans.

6. **Consume some high-quality protein at each feeding.** Fish, especially oily varieties like salmon, tuna, herring, mackerel,

sardines, and lake trout are fantastic. Other good sources are skinless poultry, beans, wild game, soy, omega-3 eggs, and shellfish. Limit red meat to two servings or less a week.

7. **Consume small, frequent meals, and *never* skip breakfast.** In contrast to those who skip breakfast, people who eat breakfast regularly significantly reduce their risk of type 2 diabetes. In addition, small frequent meals result in lower and more stable blood glucose and insulin levels over the course of the day.

8. **Consume soy foods regularly.** Soy foods have been shown to help stabilize blood glucose and insulin levels in type 2 diabetics. Make soy milk, tofu, tempeh, miso, soy nuts, and edamame a customary part of your daily fare.

9. **Take your supplements.** A multivitamin, 500-1,000 mg of vitamin C in divided doses, 400 IU of vitamin E, pharmaceutical grade fish oil, and a broad spectrum antioxidant. (See the next chapter for additional information on supplements.) If you have a chronic medical condition or take prescription drugs, consult your physician first.

10. **Regularly consume foods high in chromium: broccoli, whole grains, oysters, lobster, shrimp, mushrooms, and brewer's yeast.** Chromium is a mineral that works with insulin to transport blood glucose from the bloodstream into the cells. Inadequate levels are known to impair insulin's activity and contribute to insulin resistance, the dangerous metabolic condition precipitating type 2 diabetes.

The Biggest Killer of Them All

Heart disease is the number one killer of Americans. In 2000, the American Heart Association reported that 61 million Americans have some form of cardiovascular disease. This includes high blood pressure, coronary heart disease, and stroke. In 2000, cardiovascular disease claimed 945,836 lives, or more poignantly, it caused nearly 40 percent of all deaths in the U.S. Cardiovascular disease-related costs for 2001 were estimated at $298.2 billion.

Risk factors include:
- High blood pressure: Some 32 percent of those with high blood pressure are unaware of it.
- Tobacco use: More than 23 percent of the adult U.S. population is at increased risk due to tobacco use.
- High LDL cholesterol, low HDL cholesterol, and high triglycerides.
- Advancing age
- Family history
- Hostility/anger

- Elevated blood homocyteine level
- Sedentary lifestyle: The Centers for Disease Control and Prevention report that 75 percent of Americans do not meet the recommended daily physical activity requirements (thirty minutes a day, three to four days a week).
- Diabetes: More than 75 percent of diabetics die from heart disease or stroke.
- Obesity: Obesity is a major risk factor for heart disease.

Homocysteine—The New Cardiovascular Risk Factor

Recent studies have found that homocysteine, an amino acid metabolite, significantly increases the risk of heart attack, strokes, dementia, and possibly osteoporosis. Standard laboratory tests are now available that measure blood homocysteine levels. Levels above fifteen are considered abnormal. Consuming adequate dietary folic acid or taking a folic acid supplement (found in most multivitamins and B-complex vitamins) can reduce elevated homocysteine levels in most people. When this is not effective, the addition of vitamins B6 and B12 (found in the standard B-complex vitamin) should suffice.

---

1. **Exercise regularly for the rest of your life.** Assuming you are a non-smoker, exercise is the single most powerful step you can take to protect yourself from cardiovascular disease. (If you are a smoker, quitting is your most powerful step.) Optimally, exercise should include thirty minutes or more of aerobic activity five or more days a week.

2. **Do your fats right!** Strictly avoid trans fat, including partially hydrogenated oil, stick margarine, and shortening. In addition, reduce your intake of saturated fat by minimizing fatty cuts of beef and pork, whole dairy products, butter, palm oil, and coconut oil. Stay heart-healthy by consuming the majority of your fats from the monounsaturated oils (extra virgin olive oil, canola oil, nuts, seeds, and avocados) and foods containing omega-3 fats (salmon, tuna, herring, mackerel, sardines, walnuts, soy, flax seed, omega-3 eggs, and wheat germ).

3. **Consume seven or more servings of fruits and vegetables daily.** It is estimated that 30 percent of cardiovascular deaths are related to inadequate fruit and vegetable intake. Garlic, onions, blueberries, strawberries, red grapes, avocados, broccoli, and asparagus are especially beneficial for cardiovascular health.

4. **Do your carbs right.** Consume the majority of your carbohydrate calories from whole grains, beans/legumes, fruits, and vegetables. Minimize your intake of high glycemic index carbohydrates, such as white flour, white rice, white potatoes, and sugar. When your body is flooded with insulin in response to consuming these foods, your entire cardiovascular system suffers.

5. **Eat oily fish three or more times a week.** The omega-3 fatty acids present in oily fish protect the cardiovascular system through seven separate mechanisms.

6. **Consume nuts and seeds daily.** While walnuts and almonds seem to be the cardiovascular superstars, all nuts are great for your heart. Multiple studies have shown that 1 ounce of nuts (a small handful) eaten five or more times a week can decrease your chances of cardiovascular disease by 30-50 percent.

7. **As long as you don't have a medical condition that prohibits the use of alcohol, have a glass of red wine with your dinner.** Scores of studies have confirmed moderate drinking's ability to protect against cardiovascular disease. Additionally, red wine is loaded with heart protective antioxidant phytochemicals called flavonoids.

8. **Take your supplements and aspirin daily.** A multivitamin, 500-1,000 mg of vitamin C in divided doses, 400 IU of vitamin E, pharmaceutical grade fish oil, and a B-complex taken at the opposite end of the day from your multivitamin. (See the next chapter for additional information on supplements.) Also, take a baby aspirin (81 mg) daily. However, please consult your physician first.

9. **Strictly avoid cardiotoxic emotions.** Cardiotoxic emotions, such as anger, hostility, and depression, can elevate your cardiovascular risk. If you routinely experience these emotions, consider exploring techniques like meditation, exercise, therapy, or other stress reduction methods.

10. **Substitute soy protein for animal protein whenever possible.** Soy foods have been shown to reduce cardiovascular risk, especially when replacing saturated animal fats like red meat.

The Lyon Diet Heart Study

In 1988, French researchers studied 605 men and women who had already survived a first heart attack. The researchers put half the group on what was then the standard American Heart Association's "Heart Healthy Diet." The other half of the group was put on a Mediterranean diet. Although the study was meant to continue for five years, it was halted after two due to the profound benefits noted in the group consuming the Mediterranean diet.

Those who followed the Mediterranean diet had an unprecedented 76 percent reduced risk of death from any form of cardiovascular disease including heart attack, stroke, and heart failure. Included in the Mediterranean diet were more whole grains, an abundance of fruits and vegetables, significant amounts of fish and lean poultry, olive oil, minimal amounts of red meat, and a special margarine made of canola oil (formulated specifically for this study). In addition, those on the "Heart Healthy" diet consumed most of their fats from omega-6 fatty acids, while those on the Mediterranean diet consumed more omega-3 fatty acids.

10 STEPS TO PREVENT OR LOWER HIGH CHOLESTEROL

What You Eat Makes the Difference

High cholesterol is more directly linked to what you eat than most other diseases. We often hear how bad cholesterol is for us, but as a matter of fact, this waxy material found throughout our bodies plays an important role in making cell membranes, some hormones, and vitamin D. Cholesterol comes from two sources: the foods you eat and your body; however, it is worth noting that your liver produces all the cholesterol your body requires.

There is good cholesterol and there is bad cholesterol. Good cholesterol (HDL) removes the bad cholesterol (LDL) from your blood stream and keeps it from building up in your arteries. When too much LDL builds up on the walls of your arteries, you are at an increased risk of heart disease. This means that less blood and oxygen are getting to your heart, which can cause chest pain and heart attack. In fact, according to the National Heart, Lung, and Blood Institute's National Cholesterol Education Program, more than 90 million American adults, or about 50 percent of the adult population, have elevated blood cholesterol levels—one of the key risk factors for heart disease.

Here are the American Heart Association's recommendations regarding cholesterol:

- Your total cholesterol level should be less than 200 mg/dL. The higher your level of total cholesterol, the more likely it is that you will develop heart disease.
- Your good cholesterol level (HDL) should be 40 mg/dL or higher. A level of 60 mg/dL can help protect you from heart disease.
- Your bad cholesterol level (LDL) should be less than 130 mg/dL. (Optimally, it should less than 100.)

Fortunately, you can do something about unhealthy cholesterol levels just by changing your diet and lifestyle.

1. **Minimize saturated fats.** Saturated fat is the primary dietary culprit that elevates bad cholesterol (LDL). Saturated fats are found in fatty cuts of beef and pork, poultry skin, coconut and palm oil (regular ingredients in processed foods), and whole dairy products (whole milk, cream, whole-fat cheeses, ice cream).

2. **Strictly avoid trans fats.** Like saturated fats, trans fats elevate LDL. Additionally, they lower HDL (good cholesterol). Trans fats are found in the partially hydrogenated oils used in most commercially baked foods, such as cakes, cookies, donuts, chips, and fried fast foods. Trans fats also lurk in stick margarine and vegetable shortening.

3. **Consume as much soluble fiber as possible.** The superstar sources for soluble fiber include: whole oats, oat bran, barley, and beans. Soluble fiber is a very effective cholesterol lowering agent.

4. **Use the monounsaturated oils as your main fat source.** Extra virgin olive oil, expeller-pressed canola oil, nuts (almonds and walnuts are exceptional), and avocados have been shown to lower LDL (bad) cholesterol.

5. **Consume seven or more servings of fruits and vegetables daily.** The best fruits are oranges, blueberries, raspberries, strawberries, red grapes, apples, and pomegranates. Superstar vegetables include dark leafy greens (spinach, kale), asparagus, brussels sprouts, broccoli, and red bell peppers. Fruits and vegetables contain soluble fiber, which is known to lower LDL cholesterol levels. They're also loaded with potent antioxidants that can prevent LDL from becoming oxidized. Research indicates that LDL cholesterol is really not dangerous until it becomes oxidized.

6. **Exercise daily.** The ideal regimen is thirty minutes or more of aerobic activity five or more days a week. Regular exercise can lower LDL cholesterol levels and elevate HDL cholesterol levels, along with scores of other cardiovascular benefits.

7. **Do your carbs right by minimizing your intake of the high glycemic varieties (white flour, white rice, white potatoes, and sugar).** Replace with whole grains and beans.

8. **Substitute soy protein for animal protein as much as possible.** Try soy milk, roasted soy nuts, tofu, miso, tempeh, and edamame. Swapping soy protein for animal protein has been proven to lower LDL cholesterol levels.

9. **Use trans fat-free margarines containing plant sterols.** Try brands such as Benecol, Take Control, or Smart Balance; each is a healthy butter substitute. Plant sterols can lower bad cholesterol levels.

10. **Consume foods known to elevate your good HDL cholesterol.** These include moderate amounts of alcohol (one drink a day

for women and one to two drinks daily for men), soy foods, green tea, shiitake mushrooms, chili peppers, oily fish, olive oil, almonds, walnuts, avocados, and cooked or raw onions and garlic.

If you are male or post-menopausal, it is important to avoid iron supplements unless specifically prescribed by your physician. Excess blood iron levels can increase oxidation of LDL (bad cholesterol), and oxidized cholesterol is the form which can stick to your artery walls.

10 STEPS TO PREVENT OR LOWER HIGH BLOOD PRESSURE

Losing Weight Is Number One

Uncontrolled high blood pressure is dangerous because it can lead to stroke, heart attack, heart failure, and kidney failure. According to recent estimates, one in four U.S. adults has high blood pressure; yet, because there are no symptoms, nearly one-third of those stricken with this chronic disease are unaware they have it. This is why high blood pressure is often called the "silent killer."

Risk factors for high blood pressure include:
- · Being overweight
- · Alcohol abuse
- · High sodium diets
- · Advancing age
- · Sedentary lifestyle
- · Insulin resistance

It is wise to have your blood pressure checked frequently. Many drugstores now have accurate blood pressure testing equipment available for free. Optimal blood pressure is 115/75 or less.

Keep in mind that losing and maintaining an optimal weight is the most important strategy you can implement to combat high blood pressure, also known as hypertension.

1. **Eat as many fruits and vegetables as possible.** Countless studies have revealed that diets high in fruits and vegetables lower blood pressure and protect against hypertension. Superstar fruits for protection against high blood pressure include: red grapes, avocados, peaches, tomatoes, apricots, whole citrus, cantaloupe, and strawberries. The superstar vegetables include: spinach, collards, kale, broccoli, lima beans, soybeans, acorn squash, red and green peppers, garlic, onions, and celery.

2. **Engage in regular exercise.** Exercise is the most powerful lifestyle tool available to lower blood pressure and prevent hypertension. Strive for thirty minutes or more of moderate aerobic activity five or more days a week.

3. **Restrict alcohol consumption.** Ideally, women should have one drink or less a day, and men should have no more than two a day. Alcohol abuse is considered to be the *number one* cause of preventable hypertension.

4. **Eat potassium-rich foods daily.** These foods have been consistently linked to lower blood pressure. Superstars include: avocados, peaches, all types of tomatoes and tomato products, salmon, soybeans, apricots, oranges, spinach, almonds, and pumpkin seeds.

5. **Consume calcium-rich foods regularly.** Foods rich in calcium lower blood pressure. The winners are canned fish with bones (salmon, mackerel, sardines), skim milk (organic is best), calcium-fortified soy milk, collards, kale, broccoli, tofu, low-fat yogurt, Parmesan cheese, and legumes, such as chick peas, white beans, pinto beans, and baked beans.

6. **Minimize salt (sodium) and excessive caffeine.** If you are hypertensive, you need to be hyper-vigilant of sodium. Ideally, limit yourself to less than 3,000 mg daily. Do not salt your food, and avoid foods with high sodium content like processed foods, fast food, and salty snack foods. Get in the habit of reading labels for sodium content, too. Excessive caffeine (coffee, sodas) can elevate blood pressure in susceptible individuals. Moderate consumption (two or less cups a day) of coffee or tea is acceptable.

7. **Regularly eat fatty fish.** The best are salmon, tuna, mackerel, lake trout, sardines, and herring. The omega-3 fatty acids found in fish have been shown to reduce blood pressure along with several other cardiovascular benefits. Strive for three servings a week. Take pharmaceutical grade fish oil on the days you don't eat oily fish. (See the next chapter for additional information on supplements.)

8. **Restrict the high glycemic index carbs, such as white flour, white rice, white potatoes, and sugar.** These foods lead to rapid elevations of blood glucose and blood insulin levels, which can directly elevate blood pressure. White carbs can also predispose you to weight gain, which further elevates blood pressure.

9. **Strictly avoid cardiotoxic emotions.** Cardiotoxic emotions, such as anger and hostility, can elevate your blood pressure. If you routinely experience these emotions, consider exploring techniques like meditation, exercise, therapy, or other forms of stress reduction.

10. **Use extra virgin olive oil daily.** Many studies have shown that this simple food lowers blood pressure. Olive oil is rich in phytochemical polyphenols, antioxidant substances that can dilate arteries.

10 STEPS TO PREVENT COLON CANCER

The Importance of Diet

If there is a cancer that responds to diet and lifestyle in cause and prevention, it's colon cancer. Cancer of the colon and rectum is the third most common cancer in the U.S. In 2003, an estimated 105,500 cases of colon cancer, and 42,000 cases of rectal cancer were diagnosed. Colorectal cancer accounts for about 10 percent of all cancer-related deaths.

Being overweight or obese increases your chances of getting this deadly cancer. If you have a high-fat and/or low-fiber diet, an inadequate intake of fruits and vegetables, drink excessive alcohol, eat lots of red meat, eat lots of refined carbohydrates, or you avoid physical activity, you're at an increased risk as well.

Additional risk factors include: smoking, advancing age (90 percent of those diagnosed are over the age of fifty), a positive family history, and a history of colon polyps or inflammatory bowel disease.

The American Cancer Society recommends screening for average-risk individuals beginning at age fifty. This includes yearly fecal occult blood testing and periodic colonoscopy. How important is it to get screening tests for colorectal cancer? When this form of cancer is detected at an early stage, the five-year survival rate is 90 percent.

If you don't have a first-degree family member with colon cancer, you need to have a colonoscopy starting at age fifty and every ten years thereafter, or as directed by your physician. If you do have a family history, you need to begin screening one decade prior to when your family member was diagnosed, and continue doing so every three to five years thereafter, or as recommended by your physician.

1. **Minimize consumption of red meat.** It is best to limit beef, pork, and lamb to two servings per week or less. Numerous studies have shown a strong association between red meat consumption and an increased risk for colon cancer.

2. **Minimize or strictly avoid alcohol.** Studies show a direct association between increased alcohol consumption and increased colon cancer risk. Alcohol can lower the absorption of folate and interfere with its functioning. Low blood levels of folate are strongly implicated in increasing the risk of colon cancer. If you drink alcohol, limit yourself to one drink a day. Try to avoid beer, as it seems to be more harmful than other types of alcohol.

3. **Eat as many fruits and vegetables as possible—aim for seven servings or more daily.** Superstar vegetables for colon cancer protection include: the allium family (garlic and onions), cruciferous veggies (broccoli, brussels sprouts, cauliflower), tomatoes and tomato products (juice, sauce, ketchup, salsa), carrots, dark leafy greens (spinach, turnip greens, romaine lettuce, mustard greens), asparagus, okra, and avocados. The superstar fruits include: apples, berries, and whole citrus.

4. **Take a daily aspirin.** (Consult with your physician first.) Aspirin's anti-inflammatory effects appear to reduce the inci-

dence of colon polyps (the precursor to colon cancer). There is a wealth of scientific data that regular aspirin use can significantly reduce the risk of colon cancer. Talk to your physician about the best dose, as the ideal dose has not been firmly established yet.

5. **Do your fats right!** Strictly avoid trans fat, including partially hydrogenated oil, stick margarine, and shortening. In addition, reduce your intake of saturated fat by minimizing fatty cuts of beef and pork, whole dairy products, butter, palm oil, and coconut oil. Stay heart-healthy by consuming the majority of your fats from the monounsaturated oils (extra virgin olive oil, canola oil, nuts, seeds, and avocados) and foods containing omega-3 fats (salmon, tuna, herring, mackerel, sardines, walnuts, soy, flax seed, omega-3 eggs, and wheat germ).

6. **Minimize high glycemic index carbohydrates, such as white flour products, white rice, white potatoes, and sugars/sweets.** White carbs can lead to rapid surges in blood glucose and blood insulin levels. Elevated blood insulin levels result in hormonal changes known to stimulate growth of cancer cells.

7. **Exercise regularly for the rest of your life.** Regular exercise reduces colon cancer risk. Aim for thirty minutes or more of aerobic activity five or more days a week.

8. **Consume low-fat yogurt with live cultures regularly.** Yogurt is high in two nutrients associated with colon cancer protection: vitamin D and calcium. Yogurt with live cultures also contains beneficial bacteria like lactobacillus acidophilus and lactobacillus bifidus, which can promote the health of cells lining the colon. Try Stonyfield Farms yogurt; it is organic and contains several strains of healthy bacteria.

9. **Regularly eat beans.** Beans are uniquely high in soluble fiber and folate, as well as calcium—all of which are associated

with protection against colon cancer. Chickpeas, lentils, black beans, lima beans, and soybeans are especially beneficial.

10. **Take your supplements daily.** A multivitamin, 500-1,000 mg of vitamin C in divided doses, 400 IU of vitamin E, pharmaceutical grade fish oil, a calcium supplement containing vitamin D, and 200 mcg of the mineral selenium, or eat one to two Brazil nuts as an alternative. (See the next chapter for additional information on supplements.) If you have a chronic medical condition or take prescription drugs, consult your physician first.

> According to a study in the *Journal of the National Cancer Institute* (February 4, 2004, Volume 96 (3)), colon cancer risk increases as dietary glycemic load rises. Of the 38,000 women who participated in this Harvard based study, those with the highest glycemic diets were about three times more likely to get colon cancer versus women with the lowest glycemic diets.

The Link Between Weight and Arthritis

Osteoarthritis, or degenerative joint disease (DJD), is one of the most common forms of arthritis. This painful and frequently debilitating condition most commonly affects middle-aged to older individuals. The more than 20 million Americans who suffer from osteoarthritis experience a breakdown in the cartilage resulting in painful and swollen joints particularly of the fingers, knees, hips, and spine.

Aside from advancing age, additional risk factors for this condition include: being overweight or obese, a positive family history, previous joint injury, and vitamin D deficiency. Extensive research has conclusively linked weight gain and obesity to DJD. Carrying around excess poundage is especially damaging to the larger, weight bearing joints of the lower extremities, namely the hips and knees. Gaining just 10 pounds can increase the force these joints must bear from 25 to 100 pounds.

1. **Exercise regularly for the rest of your life.** Exercise and weight maintenance are now considered the cornerstones of therapy and prevention for this disease. Inactivity leads to inadequate flow of joint fluid, causing the cartilage to become dry and brittle, and therefore much more susceptible to damage. The movement of the joints during exercise circulates the fluid that nourishes and lubricates cartilage. Exercise strengthens the muscles, ligaments, and tendons that support the joints, thereby removing pressure or decreasing the load the joints have to bear. Range of motion and flexibility are also increased with exercise. Finally, the impact of exercise on weight loss and weight maintenance is critically important. Losing just 10 pounds can decrease the weight-bearing load of your large joints (hips and knees) from 25-100 pounds.

   For joints of the lower extremities (hips, knees, ankles, feet), walking, cycling, and water aquatics are fantastic. Use of free weights or weight machines provides the best exercise for the joints of the upper body (wrist, elbow, shoulders, spine, fingers). Regular exercise done properly has also been proven to relieve arthritis related joint pain.

2. **Minimize consumption of omega-6 oils, especially corn, safflower, sunflower, cottonseed, peanut, and soybean oil.** These oils promote inflammation in your body. Instead, use canola and olive oil; both are low in omega-6 fatty acids. Note, omega-6 oils are found in abundance in many processed foods—*check the labels!*

3. **Maximize your intake of omega-3 fats.** Consume oily fish (salmon, sardines, tuna, mackerel, anchovies, herring, lake trout), walnuts, canola oil, whole soy foods, flaxseeds, wheat germ, and omega-3 eggs. Omega-3 fatty acids, found in highest concentrations in oily fish, decrease inflammation. Inflammation is the primary cause of arthritis pain.

4. **Consume as many vegetables as possible. Aim for five or more servings a day.** Superstar vegetables for arthritis include: onions (red are best), celery, tomatoes, broccoli, brussels sprouts, red bell peppers, garlic, and dark leafy greens (watercress, spinach, kale)

5. **Eat your fruit.** Aim for two servings a day of the following superstars: apples, red grapes, blueberries, blackberries, raspberries, cranberries, cherries, oranges, and plums. Like the vegetables above, these foods contain antioxidant and anti-inflammatory compounds useful in prevention of DJD.

6. **Minimize consumption of animal products high in arachidonic acid.** Red meat, poultry skin, and whole dairy products are the richest dietary sources of this potent pro-inflammatory omega-6 fat.

7. **Spice up your food with rosemary, ginger, turmeric, and curry.** With their potent phytochemicals, these herbs and spices can help assuage arthritis pain. Opt for fresh rosemary and fresh ginger root, grated or chopped for the most anti-inflammatory punch. Curcumin, the pigment which gives turmeric and curry their brilliant yellow color, is one of the most potent natural anti-inflammatory substances known.

8. **Take your supplements daily.** A multivitamin, 500-1,000 mg of vitamin C in divided doses, 400 IU of vitamin E, and pharmaceutical grade fish oil.Consider a calcium/vitamin D supplement if you don't consume several calcium rich foods daily. (See the next chapter for additional information on supplements.) If you have a chronic medical condition or take prescription drugs, consult your physician first.

9. **Take specific joint-health supplements.** Take 1,000-2,000 mg per day of glucosamine in *sulfate* form, along with chondroitin sulfate, 800-1,600 mg per day in two divided doses. Look for these supplements in one convenient tablet. As with

many supplements, it may take up to two months of continual use to feel results.

Another popular and effective joint supplement is MSM, which is frequently found in combination with glucosamine and chondroitin. You should take 500-3,000 mg daily of MSM for best results.

10. **Sip on green or black tea daily.** Freshly brewed green and black teas are filled with joint-preserving phytochemicals. Add a small piece of freshly chopped ginger root for an incomparable joint-healthy drink.

10 STEPS TO PREVENT ALZHEIMER'S DISEASE

What You Eat Can Affect Your Mind

Alzheimer's is a debilitating disease that destroys brain cells. Although poorly understood, it is now considered the leading cause of dementia—the decline in thinking skills. Today, approximately 4.5 million Americans have been diagnosed with the disease.

Alzheimer's symptoms can include the gradual loss of memory; the inability to recognize people, places, or things; difficulty reasoning; disorientation; and the loss of language skills. According to the Alzheimer's Association, sufferers can also undergo personality changes, behavioral changes, and hallucinations.

Although scientists have not found the cause of Alzheimer's, risk factors have been identified, including advancing age, a positive family history, previous head injury with loss of consciousness, elevated blood homocysteine levels, and possibly smoking.

1.　**Maximize your intake of omega-3 fatty acids.** Consume oily fish at least three times a week (salmon, sardines, tuna, mackerel, anchovies, herring, lake trout). Also, consume walnuts, canola oil, whole soy foods, flaxseeds, wheat germ, and omega-3 eggs. Omega-3 fats comprise the majority of the solid structure of the brain. In addition, they are essential for maintenance of a healthy cardiovascular system, one of your biggest allies in protecting yourself from this devastating disease.

2. **Minimize your intake of saturated fat, and completely avoid trans fat.** Saturated fat (found in fatty cuts of beef, pork, and lamb, whole dairy products, poultry skin, and coconut and palm oil) and trans fat (found in stick margarines, partially hydrogenated oils, and most processed foods) are known to do damage to your arteries. Maintaining healthy blood flow to the brain is fundamental to protecting against Alzheimer's and requires healthy arteries.

3. **Keep your blood pressure in the optimal range of 115/75 or less.** Elevated blood pressure will impair healthy blood flow to your brain. Take a look at the 10 Steps to Prevent High Blood Pressure for more information.

4. **Exercise regularly for the rest of your life.** Regular exercise is proven to enhance brain function and promote arterial health. To prevent cognitive decline, exercise that involves some mental effort is particularly effective (for example, dancing). A number of studies are now reporting that regular exercise may protect specifically against Alzheimer's, as well as other forms of mental deterioration and dementia.

5. **Eat as many fruits and vegetables as possible; aim for seven or more a day.** Evidence is mounting that inflammation plays a fundamental role in the development of Alzheimer's. Many authorities also believe that free radical damage to vital brain structure is involved as well. The beneficial phytochemicals concentrated in fruits and vegetables provide anti-inflammatory power and can "arrest" free radicals and prevent them from damaging your cells.

The superstar fruits for Alzheimer's protection include: apples, red grapes, all berries (with blueberries at the top of the list), cherries, pomegranates, oranges, and plums. Superstar vegetables include: onions (red are best), tomatoes, broccoli, brussels sprouts, red bell peppers, garlic and dark leafy greens like watercress, kale, spinach, and collards.

6. **Take low dose aspirin or ibuprofen regularly. (Consult with your physician first.)** These over-the-counter remedies help decrease inflammation in your body and have shown scientific promise in Alzheimer's protection.

7. **Minimize foods known to promote inflammation in your body.** These include the omega-6 fats found in corn, safflower, sunflower, soybean, and cottonseed oil. Trade these in for the monounsaturated fats found in canola and olive oil. Also, avoid foods containing arachidonic acid—red meat, whole dairy, and poultry skin. Arachidonic acid is a potent, pro-inflammatory omega-6 fatty acid.

8. **Engage your brain in learning all your life.** Several studies have reported that people with the most education in their younger years are less likely to develop dementia. It's also been reported that those who regularly engage in cognitive stimulating activities, such as reading, playing cards, working crossword puzzles, and the like, have a significantly reduced risk of Alzheimer's or dementia. Learning how to play a musical instrument or how to speak a new language can offer dramatic benefits to cognitive/brain function.

9. **Consume foods rich in vitamin E regularly.** This very potent antioxidant and anti-inflammatory vitamin has been shown in compelling studies to offer significant Alzheimer's protection. As is generally the case, the best results have been with high food intakes of vitamin E. Rich sources are: nuts and seeds (especially sunflower seeds, walnuts, almonds, and hazelnuts), wheat germ, soybeans, lima beans, and bran.

10. **Take your supplements daily.** A multivitamin, 500-1,000 mg of vitamin C in divided doses, 400 IU of vitamin E, pharmaceutical grade fish oil, and a B-complex vitamin taken at the opposite end of the day from your multivitamin, which protects against an elevated homocysteine level. (See the next chapter for additional information on supplements.) If you have a chronic medical condition or take prescription drugs, consult your physician first.

DR. ANN'S GUIDE TO SUPPLEMENTS

As you know by now, I'm a huge proponent of eating all the right foods, not only to guard your health, but also as a basis to shed those unnecessary pounds. We will never be able to replace Mother Nature's ability to create foods filled with thousands of different compounds, supplying our daily needs and protecting us against diseases—but supplements do offer us yet another way to ensure our good health. Evolving medical science tells us that within our modern food culture, our chances of optimal health without the use of a few key supplements are decreasing. We have recently learned that even a marginal deficiency of certain key nutrients can significantly increase the risk of deadly diseases like cancer, heart disease, and Alzheimer's. In addition, consuming certain nutrients above the minimum daily requirement may offer added disease protection. When it comes to supplements, even the ultra-conservative American Medical Association (AMA) is firmly on record, claiming that all adults need to take a daily multivitamin. The following list of recommended supplements provides a simple, quick, safe, and cost-effective means to safeguard against nutrient deficiencies and to minimize your chances of developing certain diseases. This extra step can maximize your chances of wellness and vitality; however, if you take prescription drugs, have a chronic medical condition, or are pregnant or nursing, please check with your healthcare provider before taking any supplements.

Recommended Supplements

1. A daily multivitamin, which contains:
    - · 400 mcg folic acid (folate, a B vitamin)
    - · 2 mg vitamin B6
    - · 6 mcg vitamin B12
    - · 15 mg of zinc
    - · 400 IU of vitamin D
    - · For men and most post-menopausal women, no iron (Fe) unless you have a documented iron deficiency. Having excess iron in your bloodstream can damage your cardiovascular system.
    - · No more than 5,000 IU of native vitamin A in the form of retinol or palmitate. Taking excess vitamin A in this form may lead to birth defects in pregnant women and increase the risk of hip fracture in others.
    - · As with all supplements, for optimal absorption and utilization take with food.

    Almost any standard, iron-free multivitamin will supply these nutrients. To ensure quality, buy a reputable national brand that has the "USP" (United States Pharmacopeia) certification on its label.

2. Additional vitamin C and vitamin E

    Unfortunately, standard multivitamins rarely contain optimal levels of these important antioxidant vitamins. Please note that vitamin C and vitamin E work as a team in your body, and therefore, are best taken together.

· Vitamin C: 500-1,000 mg a day. Best taken in divided doses, morning and evening.
· Vitamin E: 400 IU a day.
· Take with food.

3.   **Long chain omega-3 fatty acids from pharmaceutical grade fish oil**

Unfortunately, the majority of Americans do not get optimal amounts of omega 3 from their diets. Certified pharmaceutical grade fish oil products ensure safety, quality, and potency. While lesser brands are considerably cheaper, they can be sources of dangerous environmental contaminants like PCBs, dioxins, and heavy metals. Still, this should not dissuade you; seek out pharmaceutical grade fish oil and take it daily. Several high-quality brands are available. You will typically only find them in health food stores or organic grocery stores. Nordic Naturals and Health from the Sun are two reputable national brands that can also be purchased online.

· Take approximately 1 gram of combined DHA/EPA daily. This is generally what's recommended on the bottle and is equivalent to the amount of long chain omega-3 fats in a modest serving of wild Alaskan salmon. To be most cost efficient, you can omit your supplement on days you have oily fish.
· Store your fish oil supplements in the refrigerator.
· If you take pharmaceutical grade fish oil supplements it's important to take 400 IU of the antioxidant vitamin E daily. Long chain omega-3 fats are prone to oxidation. Having good blood levels of vitamin E will protect these molecules from oxidative damage.
· Always take at mealtime.

4. Calcium

I recommended calcium supplements for all women who are of perimenopausal age or older. Men need only to take calcium at their physicians' recommendations. Calcium citrate is the most bioavailable form. Avoid calcium from dolomite, coral, oysters, or bone meal, as they may contain heavy metals.

- Take 1,000-1,200 mg per day.
- Take calcium in divided doses, twice a day.
- If you take supplemental calcium it's critical that you make sure you are getting adequate supplemental magnesium as well. It's best to take calcium and magnesium in a 2:1 or 3:1 ratio. In other words, if you take 1,200 mg of calcium a day, take 400-600 mg of magnesium along with it. Remember that many multivitamins contain some magnesium.
- Take calcium with food.

5. B-complex

I recommend a daily B-complex supplement for those at risk for, or diagnosed with, Alzheimer's or cardiovascular disease. Also, those who undergo chronic stress or drink alcohol daily should consider taking a B-complex supplement.

- Take one a day at the opposite time of day from your multivitamin. (For example, multivitamin in morning, B-complex at night.)
- Take your B-complex supplement with food.

6. Other Supplement Considerations

Smokers, individuals with type 2 diabetes, and people who take prescription drugs, exercise vigorously, live in areas with excessive air pollution, work outdoors, or suffer chronic emotional stress have an increased need for antioxidants. If you fall into one of these categories it is especially critical that you consume the recommended servings of vegetables and fruits. Taking additional antioxidants is also prudent. Because individual antioxidants have very specific roles in the body, and because many work synergistically with one another, it is best to take a supplement containing small amounts of lots of them in one formulation. For best results look for a supplement with several or more of the following:

· Alpha lipoic acid
· Grape seed extract
· Vitamin C
· Coenzyme CoQ10
· Pine bark extract
· Pycnogenol
· Selenium
· Green tea extract
· Bilberry
· Mixed carotenoids
· Zinc
· Rosemary
· Ginger
· Turmeric
· Glutathione
· Vegetable powder blend
· Fruit powder blend

Part 4
Sample Meal Plans
and Recipes

★ Denotes recipes contributed by celebrity chef Kevin Graham, the author of four books and previous executive chef of the famed Windsor Court Hotel in New Orleans. Renowned for excellence across the United States, Chef Kevin was voted by his peers as Best Chef in the City (New Orleans) in 1995 and named as one of the Top Ten Chefs in the USA in 1991 by *Food & Wine*.

BREAKFAST

Unsweetened coffee (black or with skim milk) or unsweetened tea as desired.

- 3/4 cup whole grain cereal of choice (see shopping list) topped with 1 Tbsp of ground flax or wheat germ, 1 Tbsp of chopped walnuts, and 1/2 cup berries of choice with 2/3 cup 1%, skim milk, or soy milk

- Caramelized Onion Omelet (see recipe)
  1/2 red grapefruit or superstar fruit of choice
  3/4 cup of V8 or tomato juice

- 1/2 cup Homemade Granola (see recipe) with 1/2 cup 1%, skim milk, or soy milk
  Orange Tossed with Mint (see recipe)

- 1 cup cooked oatmeal (slow cooking or steel cut oats are best) with 1/2 cup berries of choice or 1/4 cup chopped dried apricots, 1 Tbsp of ground flax or 1 Tbsp chopped walnuts
  3/4 cup Fresh Blended Tomato (see recipe)

- 2 slices 100% whole grain toast topped with 1 Tbsp each natural-style peanut butter or almond nut butter
  Superstar fruit of choice

- Egg White Frittata with Bell Peppers (see recipe)
  1/4 cantaloupe
  3/4 cup V8 or tomato juice

- Scrambled Omega-3 Eggs with Salsa (see recipe)
  3/4 cup V8 or tomato juice

- 3 Almond Oatmeal Pancakes (see recipe)
  Cantaloupe with Lime Juice and Dried Apricots (see recipe)

- 1/2 whole grain bagel topped with 2 slices of smoked salmon, 1 slice red onion, 1 slice tomato, 1 tsp capers, 1 Tbsp yogurt cheese
  1/2 red grapefruit

- Sautéed Spinach with Poached Omega-3 Eggs (see recipe)
  1/2 cup Blueberries in Balsamic Vinegar (see recipe)
  3/4 cup Chef Kevin's Vegetable Juice (see recipe)

- Breakfast Salad with Ricotta Cheese (see recipe)
  1 Wasa cracker with 1 Tbsp natural-style peanut butter or almond nut butter

- Omega-3 Veggie Omelet (see recipe)

- Warm Breakfast Salad (see recipe)

- Smoked Salmon Frittata (see recipe)

On the Go Breakfasts

· 1 1/2 ounces (a healthy handful) of mixed nuts or nut of
choice
1 green apple

· 1 mozzarella cheese stick
1 ounce (a small handful) nuts of choice
1 orange or superstar fruit of choice

· 8-ounce low-fat plain yogurt, sweetened with Splenda if
desired
1 ounce (a small handful) of nuts of choice
Superstar fruit of choice

· 2 hard-boiled omega-3 eggs
Superstar fruit of choice

Recipes

Caramelized Onion Omelet

Thinly slice 1 medium yellow onion and cook in skillet with 1 teaspoon canola oil until caramelized. Add 2 omega-3 eggs to create an omelet.

Serves 1

Homemade Granola

1 pound rolled oats
1 1/2 cups shelled, unsalted sunflower seeds
1 1/2 cups slivered almonds
1/4 cup shelled, unsalted pumpkin seeds
1/2 cup pine nuts
1/2 cup shelled, unsalted pistachio nuts
1/2 cup shelled pecans, roughly chopped
3/4 cup honey
1 1/2 teaspoons pure vanilla extract

Preheat oven to 325°F. Place the dry ingredients in large mixing bowl and combine well. Slowly stir in honey and vanilla, making sure that each grain is evenly coated. Spread the granola mixture on an ungreased baking sheet and bake for 20 minutes, or until grains become crisp and very lightly browned, stirring every 5 minutes to prevent granola from sticking to pan and burning. Remove the granola from the oven and allow to cool (it will become crunchier as it cools). Granola can be stored at room temperature in airtight containers or in the freezer in a plastic bag.

Makes 4 pounds

Orange Tossed with Mint

1 orange peeled, with as much of the pith removed as possible
1/2 teaspoon freshly chopped mint

Slice the orange crosswise and toss together in a bowl with 1/2 teaspoon finely chopped mint.

Serves 1

Fresh Blended Tomato

2 large ripe tomatoes washed, with eyes removed

Place the tomatoes in a high-speed blender and blend for 1 minute. Add a dash of Tabasco to spice up the flavor and serve over crushed ice with a twist of lemon.

Serves 1

Egg White Frittata with Bell Peppers

3 raw egg whites
2 tablespoons finely chopped onion
1/3 cup diced red bell pepper
1/3 cup diced green bell pepper
1/3 cup diced yellow bell pepper
1/4 jalapeno (optional)
1 tablespoon olive oil

In a nonstick pan sauté onions and peppers until soft. In a separate bowl, whip egg whites for about 1 minute, or until they start to foam. Add foamy egg whites to the peppers and onions in the pan and place in a preheated 375°F oven for about 10 minutes, or until the center of the frittata is cooked. Slide out of the pan and onto plate.

Serves 2

Scrambled Omega-3 Eggs with Salsa

1 teaspoon olive oil
2 omega-3 eggs
2 tablespoons salsa

Preheat a nonstick pan and add olive oil. Pour in the eggs and stir with a nonmetal spoon or spatula until eggs are cooked.

Serves 1

Salsa

6 Roma tomatoes
2 cloves garlic
1 jalapeno (optional)
1 red onion
Juice of one lemon and one lime
3 tablespoons chopped cilantro
3 tablespoons olive oil

Remove eyes from tomatoes and brush with olive oil. Stem the jalapeno, split down the middle, and remove seeds. Brush with oil. Halve the red onion and brush with oil, and place one half on a baking sheet and roast in a preheated oven at 375°F for 12 minutes. Remove and allow to cool. Blend ingredients quickly for about 10 seconds, or longer if you would like it smoother. Dice the remaining 1/2 onion and add chopped cilantro. Mix in a bowl with lemon and lime juices. Add it to the blended ingredients and season with salt and pepper.

Almond Oatmeal Pancakes

1/2 cup almond flour
1/2 cup oatmeal
4 omega-3 egg whites
4 ounces plain yogurt
Pinch of salt
Cooking spray

Combine ingredients in a blender and blend for 2 minutes. In a nonstick pan, lightly spray the inner surface and using a 2 ounce ladle, place the amount in the pan and cook until brown on one side and then flip. Serve hot.

Serves 4

Cantaloupe with Lime Juice and Dried Apricots

1/4 cantaloupe, skinned and seeds removed
Juice of one fresh lime
2 tablespoons dried apricots, finely chopped

In a bowl, combine all ingredients and allow to sit for 20 minutes so the apricots can reconstitute a little.

Serves 1

Sautéed Spinach with Poached Eggs

10 cups spinach washed and diced
1 French shallot, finely minced
1 small pinch of nutmeg
1 teaspoon grated Parmesan
2 poached omega-3 eggs
1 pint water
2 tablespoons of vinegar

In a heavy pan, bring water and vinegar to a rolling boil. With a spoon, stir the water to create a whirlpool. Drop the eggs into the center and bring the heat down to a simmer, cook for about 3-4 minutes. With a slotted spoon, remove the eggs and drain on kitchen paper.

In a sauté pan, cook the shallot in olive oil until translucent. Add the spinach, stirring slowly until wilted. Add the nutmeg and remove from heat. Drain into a colander and press spinach with a spoon to remove excess water. Place the spinach on a plate, place the poached egg on top, and sprinkle with Parmesan. Serve hot.

Serves 1

Blueberries in Balsamic Vinegar

1 pint blueberries, washed and diced
2 tablespoons balsamic vinegar

In a nonstick pan bring the vinegar to a boil. Add the blueberries and remove from heat after about 15 seconds. The blueberries should bloom (swell). Serve right away.

Serves 2

Chef Kevin's Vegetable Juice

1 cucumber, washed and peeled
1 carrot
1 broccoli head
3 celery stalks
6 large ripe tomatoes
3 large oranges, washed and diced
1 bunch of parsley

Combine all ingredients and blend until smooth. Strain and serve.

4-6 Servings

Breakfast Salad with Ricotta Cheese

1/4 cup raspberries, washed and diced
1/4 cup strawberries, washed and diced
1/4 cup blueberries
1/4 cup ricotta cheese, drained
1/4 cup dried apricots
1/4 teaspoon chopped mint
1/4 teaspoon chopped basil
1/4 teaspoon chopped dill

Mix all ingredients together in a bowl and serve right away.

Serves 2

Omega-3 Eggs Veggie Omelet

2 omega-3 eggs
3 superstar veggies of choice (about 1 cup total) sautéed in 1
teaspoon canola oil
1/4 cup shredded part-skim mozzarella cheese

Serves 1

Warm Breakfast Salad

4 cups baby spinach leaves sautéed with 1 teaspoon olive oil and 1 clove minced garlic. Top with 1 sliced hard-boiled omega-3 egg, 2 slices chopped Canadian bacon, 1 tablespoon crumbled feta cheese.

Serves 1

Smoked Salmon Frittata

4 omega-3 eggs
2 tablespoons chopped red onion
3 ounces smoked salmon, chopped
1 tablespoon capers
1 tablespoon extra virgin olive oil

In nonstick skillet, sauté onions in olive oil until soft. Stir in the capers and salmon. Add beaten eggs. Cover and cook over medium to low heat for about 8 minutes or until the bottom is set and the top is slightly undercooked. Put in preheated broiler until the top is set.

Serves 2

LUNCH

- Broccoli Florets with Lemon Manchego Cheese (see recipe)
  Mixed Leaves with Basil Mint and Cilantro and Grilled
  Chicken Breast (see recipe)

- PB&J (see recipe)
  1 green apple

- 3/4 cup low-fat cottage cheese mixed with 1/2 cup berries of
  choice
  2 Wasa whole grain crackers topped with 1 teaspoon each of
  peanut butter or other nut butter

- Salad du Jour (see recipe)

- Homemade Veggie Pizza (see recipe)

- Tuna on Rye (see recipe) or tuna stuffed in a cored tomato
  1/2 avocado sliced with fresh lemon juice

- Avocado and Tomato Salad with Feta Cheese (see recipe)
  Seared Tuna with Hummus Dip (see recipe)

- Tempeh/Veggie Wrap (see recipe)
  1 part-skim mozzarella cheese stick

- Romaine Lettuce and Watercress with Cucumber Dressing
  (see recipe)
  Lentils with Salmon Cubes (see recipe)

- Curried Salmon Salad on Toasted Sourdough (see recipe) or
  placed in cored red bell pepper
  1/2 cup baby carrots drizzled with Balsamic vinegar

- Broiled Chicken Breast with Cashews and Cauliflower
  (see recipe)
  Small Tossed Salad (see recipe)

- Turkey Wrap (see recipe)
  1/2 red bell pepper cut into slices and dipped in hummus

- Turkey Burger All the Way (see recipe)
  1/2 sliced orange bell pepper drizzled with Balsamic vinegar

- Roast Beef and Swiss Pita Sandwich (see recipe)

- Spinach Salad with Almonds and Shredded Carrots (see
  recipe)

Recipes

Broccoli Florets with Lemon Manchego
★ Cheese
★ ★

> 1 cup of broccoli florets washed
> 1/4 cup of lemon juice
> 1/8 cup of pumpkin seed oil
> 1/3 cup grated Manchego cheese

Combine all ingredients in a bowl and mix well.

Serves 2

★ Mixed Leaves with Grilled Chicken
★ ★

> 2 chicken breasts
> 1 egg white
> 2 teaspoons curry powder
> Cooking spray
> 2 cups mixed lettuce leaves
> 1 cup bean sprouts
> 1/4 cup basil, roughly chopped
> 1/4 cup mint leaves
> 1/4 cup cilantro
> 2 tablespoons of Tamari Soy
> 1 tablespoon sesame oil

Combine mixed lettuce leaves and all subsequent ingredients in a bowl and mix. Divide into 2 plates.

Marinate the chicken with egg whites for 20 minutes then wash off the whites and dry. Preheat the grill or broiler. Dust the chicken with curry powder on both sides. Spray pan with nonstick pan spray; place on grill, or under broiler in a sturdy pan. Cook on both sides turning regularly for 12-15 minutes. Place on a bed of greens.

Serves 2

PB&J

2 tablespoons natural-style peanut butter or other nut butter
1 tablespoon spreadable fruit
2 slices of 100% whole grain bread

Serves 1

Salad du Jour

2 cups dark salad greens of choice
2 or more 1/2 cup servings chopped superstar vegetables of choice
1 tablespoon nuts/seeds of choice
3 ounces of lean meat (skinless turkey, chicken, or fresh ham) or fish of choice
2 tablespoons vinaigrette of choice (see recipes)

Serves 1

Quick Homemade Veggie Pizza

1 whole grain tortilla or 1 slice whole grain pita
3 tablespoons tomato sauce
1 cup baby spinach leaves
3 tablespoons canned roasted red peppers
1 tablespoon pine nuts
1 tablespoon chopped fresh basil
1/2 cup shredded part-skim mozzarella cheese
1 clove minced garlic
1 tablespoon balsamic vinaigrette (see recipe)

Spread tomato sauce over tortilla, top with spinach, garlic, peppers, pine nuts, basil, cheese, and drizzled balsamic vinaigrette. Cook at 375°F until cheese melts and spinach wilts.

Serves 1

Tuna on Rye

3 ounces canned tuna in water
1 1/2 tablespoons light mayo (or 2 tablespoons yogurt cheese)
2 tablespoons chopped yellow onion
2 tablespoons chopped celery
1 teaspoon Dijon mustard

Serves 1

★ Avocado and Tomato Salad with Feta Cheese
★
★

1 heart romaine lettuce, torn up, not cut
1 large beefsteak tomato, washed and diced
1 avocado, peeled and diced
2 tablespoons feta cheese crumbled
2 tablespoon olive oil
1/2 crushed garlic clove
2 tablespoons sherry vinegar

Combine all ingredients in a bowl and mix well. Serve immediately.

Serves 2

★ Seared Tuna with Hummus Dip
★
★

1 six-ounce tuna steak, seasoned with salt and pepper

Preheat a heavy skillet until smoking hot. Spray the tuna with pan spray and place in the skillet. Sear rapidly until a crust is formed. Flip and repeat. Cut the tuna into bite size pieces and serve with a large dollop of hummus dip.

Serves 2

Tempeh/Veggie Wrap

3 ounces crumbled soy tempeh
1 1/2 tablespoons balsamic vinaigrette
1/2 cup baby spinach leaves
1 tablespoon chopped purple onion
2 tablespoon chopped seeded cucumber
1 tablespoon sunflower seeds

Take 3 ounces crumbled soy tempeh and mix with 1 1/2 tablespoon of balsamic vinaigrette. Place with remaining ingredients in whole grain tortilla, spread with 1 1/2 tablespoons of yogurt cheese. Fold into a wrap.

Serves 1

Romaine Lettuce and Watercress with Cucumber Dressing

1 heart of romaine, washed and dried
1 bunch watercress
1 cucumber, peeled and seeded
6 mint leaves
1 cup fat-free plain yogurt

Tear the romaine lettuce and watercress and place in a bowl. In a blender place the cucumber, mint, and yogurt. Blend at high speed for 1 minute then mix with the lettuce and watercress and serve.

Serves 2

Lentils with Salmon Cubes

2 four-ounce salmon fillets, skinless and cut into 6 pieces each
1 cup cooked lentils
1 tablespoon olive oil
1 garlic clove, finely minced
1 pint of chicken or vegetable stock
Salt and pepper to taste

To cook the lentils, place them in a nonstick pan. Over a medium flame, gently toast the lentils and gradually add the chicken stock until the lentils are cooked. Season and put aside.

In a nonstick pan, place the olive oil and bring up to medium heat. Put the cubed salmon in the oil and add the garlic. Sauté for about 3-4 minutes. Season with salt and pepper.

Drain the lentils and place a generous spoonful on a plate and top with the cooked salmon and serve.

Serves 2

Curried Salmon Salad on Toasted Sourdough

3 ounces canned Wild Alaskan salmon
1 tablespoon light mayo (or 2 tablespoons yogurt cheese)
1 tablespoon chopped purple onion
1/4 teaspoon curry powder
1 tablespoon chopped celery
1 teaspoon lemon juice or Dijon mustard

Blend all ingredients and serve as a sandwich with 2 thin slices of toasted sourdough bread or whole grain bread of choice.

Serves 1

Broiled Chicken Breast with Cashews and Cauliflower

2 skinless chicken breasts
3/4 cup cauliflower florets
1/4 cup chopped cashews
1/4 cup chopped onion
1/4 teaspoon of canola oil

Place the chicken breast on a pan for broiling. Season with 2 teaspoons of canola oil and turmeric. Mix together and rub the mixture on both sides of the breast and sprinkle with salt and pepper. Place the chicken under a preheated broiler and cook on both sides approximately 7 minutes per side. Remove when cooked.

In a nonstick pan, bring the oil to medium heat and sauté the cauliflower and onions together for about 3-4 minutes then add the cashews. Divide into 2 plates, place the chicken on top and serve.

Serves 2

Small Tossed Salad

Mixed greens
Red and orange bell peppers
Cherry tomatoes
Cucumbers
1-2 tablespoon vinaigrette of choice (see recipes)

Serves 1

Turkey Wrap

3 ounces thinly sliced turkey
1 teaspoon Dijon mustard
1/2 tablespoon light mayo (or 1 tablespoon yogurt cheese)
2 slices purple onion
2 slices tomato
1/2 cup chopped lettuce

Place on a whole grain tortilla and fold into a wrap.

Serves 1

Turkey Burger All the Way

1 four-ounce patty of skinless ground turkey breast
1 whole grain bun
1 slice red onion
2 romaine lettuce leaves
1 slice tomato
1 teaspoon Dijon mustard
1 tablespoon ketchup
1 slice reduced-fat cheddar cheese

Serves 1

Roast Beef and Swiss Pita Sandwich

3 ounces lean deli-style roast beef

1/2 cup shredded lettuce

2 slices tomato

1 slice purple onion

1 teaspoon Dijon mustard

1 tablespoon yogurt cheese mixed with 1/4 teaspoon prepared horseradish

1 slice reduced-fat Swiss cheese

1 slice whole grain pita

Serves 1

Spinach Salad with Almonds and Shredded Carrots

4 cups spinach washed and diced

1 tablespoon slivered almonds

1 small carrot shredded

2 tablespoons olive oil

1 teaspoon balsamic vinegar

1 teaspoon toasted pumpkin seeds

Combine all ingredients and toss with oil and vinegar, serve right away.

Serves 1

DINNER

When creating your dinner menu, don't overlook simple dishes, such as steamed broccoli, roasted vegetables, or a mixed salad of baby greens.

- Fricassee of Shrimp with Teardrop Tomatoes and Tarragon (see recipe)
  Tossed Italian Salad (see recipe)
  1/2 cup whole grain couscous

- Marinated Grilled Flank Steak with Seared Peppers (see recipe)
  Mixed salad of baby greens
  Roasted Asparagus (see recipe)

- Pork Tenderloin with Apples and Dried Apricots (see recipe)
  Mixed salad of baby greens
  Roasted Cauliflower (see recipe)

- Medallions of Veal with Celeriac and Apples (see recipe)
  Roasted Brussels Sprouts and Shallots (see recipe)
  1/2 cup brown rice

- Pan Roasted Quails with Red Cabbage and Honey Vinegar (see recipe)
  Roasted Asparagus (see recipe)
  1/2 cup whole grain couscous

- Grilled Chicken Breasts with Miso Sauce (see recipe)
  Braised Kale (see recipe)

- Seared Tenderloin with Red Pepper Hash (see recipe)
  Baby Spinach Salad (see recipe)
  1/2 cup Lentils (see recipe) or beans of choice

- Shredded Lamb with Basil and Dried Tomato (see recipe)
  Roasted Cauliflower (see recipe)
  Tossed Italian Salad (see recipe)

- Boneless Skinless Trout in Oatmeal (see recipe)
  Sautéed Medley of Peppers (see recipe)

- Lamb Chops with Curry and Peanut Sauce (see recipe)
  Edamame (see recipe)
  Tossed salad of baby mixed greens

- Grilled Snapper or Grouper with Fresh Orange and Cantaloupe (see recipe)
  Roasted Brussels Sprouts and Shallots (see recipe)
  1/2 cup black beans

- Marinated Seared Chicken Breast (see recipe)
  Roasted Cauliflower (see recipe)
  Steamed broccoli

· Pan Seared Codfish with Porcini Mushrooms and Grilled Radicchio (see recipe)
Lentils (see recipe)

· Salmon Cakes with Cucumber Dill Sauce (see recipe)
Oriental Cabbage Salad (see recipe)

Dinner Recipes

Fricassee of Shrimp with Teardrop Tomatoes and Tarragon

24 uncooked large shrimp (size equal to about 15 shrimp to the pound), peeled and de-veined
1 pint of teardrop or cherry tomatoes, washed and dried
1 red onion, finely diced
1 clove garlic, finely minced
1 teaspoon fresh tarragon leaves, finely chopped
1/4 cup of dry white wine or Pernod
4 tablespoons of canola oil

In a heavy skillet bring the olive oil up to high heat without burning it. Add the shrimp and sauté until seared on all sides. Remove from the skillet and drain. Keep the skillet on the heat, add the onion, and cook until soft. Add the garlic and tomatoes and cook until the tomatoes start to burst. Add the white wine or Pernod and tarragon. Bring to a boil and add the shrimp and simmer for about 3 minutes. Adjust the seasoning and serve.

Serves 4

Marinated Grilled Flank Steak with Seared
Peppers

1 flank steak
2 garlic cloves
1 teaspoon pepper flakes
1/2 cup lime juice
1 cup canola oil
1 chipotle pepper, finely minced
1 teaspoon coarse black pepper
1 teaspoon Herbes de Provence
1/4 cup Worcestershire

Combine all the ingredients for the marinade and mix well. In a flat casserole, cover the flank steak with the marinade and allow to sit overnight.

Preheat your grill.

Sear the flank steak on both sides, cook until medium, brushing continuously with the marinade. Remove from grill and allow to rest.

Serves 4

Seared Peppers

1 red, 1 yellow, and 1 green bell pepper, deseeded and finely sliced
1 red onion, peeled and finely sliced
4 tablespoons of the marinade (above)
Salt and pepper to taste

Mix all of the ingredients in a bowl. Lay out a large square of aluminum foil and place the mixture in the middle of the lining. Bring the four corners to the center to form a pouch and place on the grill. Cook for about 20 minutes. Serve with the sliced flank steak.

Serves 4

Pork Tenderloin with Apples and Dried Apricot

1 pork tenderloin, peeled and cleaned
2 Granny Smith apples, peeled, cored, and dried
1/2 cup dried apricots, finely diced
1 teaspoon finely chopped fresh ginger

In a bowl, combine the apple, apricots, and ginger. Mix well and allow to stand. The liquid from the apples will partially hydrate the dried apricots.

Preheat oven to 425°F. On a baking rack, season the pork tenderloin with oil, black pepper, and a little salt. Place in preheated oven for 10 minutes, then reduce the temperature to 350°F and cook until done (approx. 15-17 minutes). Remove from oven and allow to rest. Slice and serve with apples and apricots.

Serves 4

Medallions of Veal with Celeriac and Apples

2 eggs, beaten well with 1/2 cup skim milk
8 two-ounce medallions of veal (ask your butcher to cut them from the loin or the top round)
1/2 cup Parmesan
1 celeriac root, washed peeled and shredded
2 Granny Smith apples, peeled, seeded, and shredded
1/2 cup fat-free plain yogurt
Juice of 1/2 lemon
1 teaspoon chopped fresh dill
1/2 cup plain flour, seasoned with salt and pepper, for dusting. (This flour is just for dusting; do not use all of it.)
1/4 cup of olive oil
Salt and pepper to taste

In a bowl, combine the eggs and cheese. Dust the veal medallions with the seasoned flour and dip into mixture.

In a preheated pan, place the olive oil and bring up to medium heat. Lay the coated medallions down into the pan and cook until golden brown on one side, flip and repeat. Remove from pan and drain onto kitchen paper.

In a bowl combine the celeriac, apple, yogurt, dill, and lemon juice and mix well.

Serve with the veal medallion.

Serves 4

Pan Roasted Quails with Red Cabbage and Honey Vinegar

8 boneless quails
2 tablespoons olive oil
Pinch of cayenne
Salt and pepper to taste
1/2 teaspoon finely chopped thyme
1/2 teaspoon finely chopped rosemary
1 head of red cabbage, finely shredded
1 apple, peeled, cored and finely shredded
1/4 cup cider vinegar
1/2 cup honey
1 red onion, peeled and shredded
Salt and pepper

In a heavy skillet, sauté the cabbage and apples in the olive oil. Add the vinegar and honey after about 10 minutes. Cook until the cabbage is soft, stirring frequently. When cooked remove from heat and keep warm.

In a heavy skillet, bring the olive oil up to medium heat. Season the quail inside and out with the mixture of thyme, rosemary, salt and pepper, and cayenne. Place in the skillet and sear on both sides quickly. Place the skillet in a preheated 375°F oven for about 10 minutes. Remove and drain on kitchen paper and serve with the red cabbage.

Serves 4

Grilled Chicken Breasts with Miso Sauce

6 boneless chicken breasts
4 egg whites
1 tablespoon freshly ground black pepper
Pinch of salt
1 small garlic clove, peeled and minced
1 tablespoon minced fresh cilantro leaves
1 teaspoon lemon juice
2 tablespoons peanut oil
1 teaspoon toasted sesame seeds
Miso sauce

Place the chicken breasts in a mixing bowl, cover with the egg whites, and marinate for about 1 hour. (This process will plump up the breasts so that they will not dry out during cooking.)

In a small bowl, combine the pepper, salt, garlic, cilantro, lemon juice, and 1 tablespoon of the oil and mix to a paste. Remove the breasts from the egg whites, rinse under cold running water, and pat dry on kitchen towels. Brush each breast with the paste on the side of the breast. Set in a clean dish.

Bring a grill or griddle up to a high temperature (coals on a grill should be grayish white and the griddle should be just below smoking). Brush each breast with a small amount of the remaining paste, then place on the grill or griddle, seasoned side down. Cook slowly for about 5 minutes, then turn and cook an additional 5 minutes on the second side. Remove the breasts from the grill, sprinkle with the sesame seeds, and serve hot with Miso sauce.

Serves 4

Miso Sauce

1 tablespoon arrowroot
2 tablespoons rice wine vinegar
1 tablespoon peanut oil
2 cloves garlic, peeled and minced
1 cup red miso paste (available at Japanese food stores)
3 cups chicken stock
1 teaspoon tamari
4 scallions, whites and greens, finely minced
1/4 cup firm tofu, cut into 1/4-inch cubes
Pinch of red pepper flakes

In a small dish, mix the arrowroot and vinegar into a loose paste. Set aside.

Heat the oil in a large, heavy saucepan over medium-high heat. Add the garlic and sauté for 1 minute or until just softened, but not browned. Add the miso paste and stir. Add the chicken stock and bring to a simmer. Fold in the tamari and scallions and stir well. Gradually stir the arrowroot past into the simmering stock, until the stock is thick enough to coat the back of a spoon (it may not be necessary to add all of the arrowroot paste). Remove the pan from the heat and fold in the tofu and red pepper flakes. Cover and keep warm until ready to serve.

Serves 4

Seared Tenderloin with Red Pepper Hash

4 two- to three-ounce beef tenderloin steaks
1 large red bell pepper, seeded and finely chopped
1 large white onion, peeled and finely sliced
1 clove garlic, crushed
4 tablespoons olive oil
Pinch of cumin
Pinch of coriander
Salt and pepper to taste
1/4 cup sherry

In a preheated skillet, add the olive oil, season the steaks with the salt, pepper, cumin, and coriander, and sear on both sides. Remove the steaks from the skillet, keeping warm, add the peppers, cook for about 2 minutes. Add the onions and garlic, cook for a further 3 minutes. Add the sherry and reduce the sauce for another 2 minutes. Adjust the seasoning and serve with the seared steaks.

Serves 4

Shredded Lamb with Basil and Dried Tomato

1 pound of lamb, finely shredded (ask your butcher to remove all
the sinews and fat before he shreds the lamb)
2 large garlic cloves, finely minced
2 tablespoons finely shredded basil
3 tablespoons of finely minced dried tomatoes
4 tablespoons of the oil from the dried tomatoes
Salt and pepper to taste

In a bowl, combine the above ingredients and mix well. Preheat a heavy skillet, covering the base of the skillet with the mixture. Cook on high heat until a little brown. Flip as you would a pancake and repeat until brown on both sides. Remove from the pan and serve with a tappenade and toasted pita.

Serves 4

Tappenade

1 clove garlic, chopped
1 3/4 cups whole, pitted kalamata olives
2-ounce can of anchovy fillets, rinsed
2 tablespoons capers
1 teaspoon finely chopped parsley
1 teaspoon chopped fresh rosemary
3 tablespoons lemon juice
4 tablespoons olive oil

Combine garlic, olives, anchovies, capers, thyme, rosemary, and lemon juice in an electric blender. Slowly drip the olive oil into the blender while you are blending the ingredients together. Blend until a paste is formed.

Serves 4

Boneless Skinless Trout in Oatmeal

4 fish = 8 fillets of Rainbow Trout skinned and de-boned
2 cups of ground oatmeal (if you cannot find ground oatmeal,
you can grind your own in a domestic blender, don't put too
many in at once, as they tend to clog—after grounding place in
bowl.)
2 eggs beaten in a bowl
1 cup whole wheat flour in a bowl
1/3 cup olive oil
1/3 cup canola oil

Preheat a heavy skillet with the oil mixture.

Dust each fillet with flour. Then dip into the beaten egg, and coat with the ground oatmeal. Place into the hot skillet, and cook for about 3 minutes on one side or until golden brown. Flip the fillets, and repeat when cooked. Remove and drain in paper towel. Serve with fresh orange segments

Serves 4

Lamb Chops with Curry and Peanut Sauce

8 lamb chops (1 whole rack of lamb)
1 tablespoon of curry powder
2 tablespoons of canola oil

Trim as much of the fat from the chops as possible. Preheat a skillet. Dust the lamb chops with the curry powder and place in the skillet. Cook over medium heat for about 4 minutes on each side. Remove and drain on kitchen paper. Serve with the peanut sauce.

Serves 4

Peanut Sauce

1 tablespoon Smart Balance margarine
2 garlic cloves, crushed
2 French shallots, finely diced
1/4 pint warm water
2 tablespoons of soy sauce
2 tablespoons smooth peanut butter (organic)
1 teaspoon grated ginger
3 dashes hot chili sauce
1 tablespoon finely chopped cilantro

In a saucepan, melt the Smart Balance with shallots and garlic, cook until soft. Add the water, soy sauce, peanut butter, and ginger. Bring to a simmer. Add the hot chili sauce and cilantro. Remove from heat and serve.

Grilled Snapper or Grouper with Fresh Orange and Cantaloupe

4 six-ounce fish fillets
1/4 cup fresh lime juice
6 crushed black peppercorns
2 oranges, peeled with pits removed
1/2 cantaloupe, peeled and seeded
1 tablespoon minced mint leaves
3 tablespoons of canola oil

In a bowl, marinate the fish for about 3 hours in the lime juice, black pepper, and canola oil.

Preheat your grill or broiler, making sure it is very hot. Remove the fish from the marinade. (There should be enough oil to ensure that the fish does not stick; if you are unsure, spray with Pam.) If broiling, place on a small baking sheet and cook until the fish is emitting a clear juice. If grilling, ensure the grill is very hot. Place the fish on the grill and allow to cook on one side for at least 5 minutes. Flip the fish and finish. Serve with the orange and melon.

Serves 4

Marinated Seared Chicken Breast

*4 skinless chicken breasts, trimmed with the center cartilage
removed*
4 raw egg whites, lightly beaten
1 tablespoon Hungarian paprika
2 tablespoons olive oil
Salt and pepper

Marinate the chicken breast in the egg whites for 2 hours.
Remove, wash, and pat dry.

In a heave skillet, bring the olive oil up to a medium-high heat.
Dust the chicken breast with paprika and season with salt and
pepper. Place in the skillet and cook gently until done. When the
breasts plump up, they should be cooked. Remove from the pan
and serve with spinach.

Serves 4

Pan Seared Codfish with Porcini Mushrooms and Grilled Radicchio

4 codfish fillets
1 pint 1% milk
1 teaspoon chipotle paste

Mix the chipotle paste with milk. Place the cod fillets in the
milk and chipotle peppers and marinate for about 2 hours. Remove
and wash quickly under cold water to remove the milk. The marinade should have permeated between the muscles of the fish.

Preheat the grill or broiler and cook the fish as quickly as
possible. (It's okay to leave the fish a little rare.) Serve with the
porcinis and the grilled radicchio.

Serves 4

★ Grilled Radicchio

2 whole radicchios, cut in quarters with root intact
1/2 cup balsamic vinegar
1/2 cup olive oil
1 tablespoon brown sugar

In a small saucepan, warm the vinegar and dissolve sugar into it. When dissolved, add the olive oil. In a bowl, marinate the radicchio with the mixture, ensuring you get as much as possible between the leaves, and allow to sit for 2 hours.

Preheat the grill or broiler and place the radicchios either under the broiler on a tray, or directly on the grill bar. Cook for about 3 minutes, or until the radicchio has wilted. Remove and serve while still hot.

Serves 4

Sautéed Porcini Mushrooms

When shopping for porcini mushrooms, take a moment to make sure that their weight is fairly heavy relative to their size. Next, check for worms by breaking open one of the caps. If worms are present, they will be easy to spot. If porcinis are not available, substitute chanterelles.

1 pound fresh porcini mushrooms
1 tablespoon extra virgin olive oil
2 shallots, peeled and finely chopped
2 tablespoons dry white wine or vermouth
Salt to taste
Freshly ground black pepper to taste
1 tablespoon finely chopped fresh, flat-leaf parsley for garnish

Trim and discard the base of the porcini stems. Wash the mushrooms to remove any grit, then dry. Cut the caps into 1/8-inch slices.

Heat the oil in a heavy skillet over moderately high heat. Add the shallots and sauté, stirring constantly, until translucent, about 2 minutes. Add the mushrooms and cook for an additional 2 minutes, until they begin to soften. Stir in the wine, season with salt and pepper, and cook for 1 minute.

Remove the mushrooms from the pan and divide among the portions of fish. Garnish with chopped parsley and serve immediately.

Serves 4

★ Salmon Cakes with Cucumber Dill Sauce
★ ★

2 cans of Red Sockeye salmon in water, drained and flaked into
bowl
2 egg yolks
1 tablespoon Japanese bread crumbs
1 tablespoon Parmesan cheese
Salt and pepper
Canola oil

Combine all the ingredients and allow to stand for 1 hour in the refrigerator (this allows time for the breadcrumbs to soak up any excess liquid). Divide into cakes, place into a skillet with preheated oil and sauté on both sides until golden brown.

Serves 4

★ Cucumber Dill and Yogurt Dip
★ ★

1 cup European cucumber, peeled, seeded, and sliced thinly
1/4 cup plain low-fat yogurt
2 tablespoons finely chopped dill
1 tablespoon finely chopped mint

Place the sliced cucumber in a bowl and dust with salt. Allow to stand 20 minutes, then wash well under cold running water for 5 minutes. Drain well and pat dry under kitchen towels.

Combine the cucumber and the rest of the ingredients, chill and serve with the salmon cakes.

Serves 4

Oriental Cabbage Salad

1 cup cooked soba noodles
2 cups shredded Napa Cabbage
1 cup shredded white cabbage
1 cup shredded red cabbage
1 teaspoon sesame seeds
3 tablespoons rice wine vinegar
2 tablespoons honey
2 tablespoons canola oil
1 teaspoon sesame oil
Salt and pepper to taste
1/2 cup slivered almonds, toasted
4 spring onions, finely sliced
1/4 cup fresh orange juice

In a bowl, mix all the cabbage noodles and sesame seeds. In a separate bowl, combine the rest of the ingredients to form the dressing. Mix with the cabbage and serve.

Serves 4

★ Roasted Cauliflower
★ ★

1 medium head cauliflower, washed with leaves removed and cut
into fourths
1 tablespoon olive oil
1/4 teaspoon salt and white pepper
2 tablespoons white wine vinegar or cider vinegar

In a bowl, gently mix the cauliflower with the seasoning and place onto a baking sheet. Place the cauliflower into a preheated 400-degree oven, roast for about 15-20 minutes, turning the cauliflower every 5 minutes. Remove from the oven, and sprinkle the vinegar evenly over the cauliflower while still hot. Serve immediately.

Serves 4

★ Roasted Asparagus
★ ★

1 bunch green asparagus washed and trimmed at the base,
removing any dry stem
4 tablespoons olive oil
2 tablespoons balsamic vinegar
2 tablespoons minced garlic clove
Salt and pepper to taste

In a bowl, toss all the ingredients together. Preheat oven to 450 degrees. Place asparagus on a baking sheet, cook for about 12 minutes. Remove from the oven and serve with any residue from the pan drizzled over the asparagus.

Serves 4

Roasted Brussels Sprouts and Shallots

1 pound brussels sprouts, washed and with any brown or yellow leaves removed
8 ounces fresh shallots, peeled and cut into halves through the root
1 tablespoon canola oil
1/4 teaspoon sea salt
1/4 teaspoon black pepper

With a sharp knife, make a deep incision across the root of each sprout. In a bowl, mix all of the ingredients then place on a baking sheet. In a 350-degree preheated oven, cook for about 15 minutes, turning frequently. Remove from the oven and serve.

Serves 4

Braised Kale

8 cups firmly packed, stemmed, torn, and washed kale
1 large white onion, peeled and finely sliced
3 garlic cloves, finely minced
Salt and pepper
2 cups chicken stock
2 tablespoons olive oil

In a heavy skillet over high heat, sauté the onions and garlic in the olive oil and cook for 2 minutes. Add the kale to the pan, and sauté for another 2 minutes. Add the stock and the salt and pepper, cook for about 3 minutes, or until the kale is tender. Remove from the heat, drain in a colander and serve.

Serves 4

Baby Spinach, Feta, Pine Nuts, and Strawberry Salad

2 bags of baby spinach, washed and dried
2 pints strawberries, washed and stemmed (cut 1 pint into quarters)
1 cup crumbled feta cheese
1/4 cup canola oil
1/4 cup toasted pine nuts

In a bowl, toss the spinach, cut strawberries, pine nuts, and feta cheese together. In a separate bowl, crush the remaining strawberries and add oil. Gently fold the mixture into the spinach salad. Serve immediately.

Serves 4

Edamame

8 ounces of cooked edamame beans
1 box sprouts, radish, pea, or mung bean of your choice
1/2 teaspoon sesame oil
2 tablespoons saki
1 teaspoon Zamori soy
1/2 cup of shredded daikon
1 tablespoon rice wine vinegar
1 pinch coriander
1 pinch ground ginger

Combine all ingredients.

Serves 4

Sautéed Medley of Peppers

1 yellow, 1 red, 1 orange, and 1 Poblano bell pepper
1 red onion, peeled and finely sliced
1 small garlic clove
3 tablespoons olive oil
Pinch of cumin
Pinch of coriander

Clean the peppers. If you have a gas range, place the peppers directly on the burner, so that the flame can char the skin black. When the skin is black, place the peppers into a bowl and cover them with plastic film. Let the peppers sit until cold. Remove from the bowl and remove skins with a sharp knife. Remove the seeds and the stems, then slice into 1/4-inch strips.

If you do not have a gas range, rub the peppers with a little oil and roast in a 500-degree oven for about 10 minutes, then clean as above.

In a heavy skillet, sauté the onion, garlic, and cumin on high heat for about 1 minute. Add the sliced peppers and toss quickly to reheat. Season and serve.

Serves 4

Lentils

1 1/2 cups lentils
2 tablespoons canola oil
1 large carrot, peeled and finely diced
1 large yellow onion, peeled and finely diced
1 large clove garlic, peeled and minced
1 medium bay leaf
5 cups chicken stock
1/4 teaspoon freshly ground black pepper
Salt to taste

Place the lentils in a colander and pick over to remove any stones or foreign objects. Rinse under cold running water until the water runs clear.

Heat the oil in a heavy stock pot. Add the carrot, onion, garlic, and bay leaf. Sauté over low heat for about 5 minutes, or until soft. Add the lentils and chicken stock to the pot and bring to a boil. Reduce the heat to a simmer, cover and cook for 20-25 minutes, or until the lentils are tender throughout but still hold their shape. Remove from the heat. Season and serve.

Serves 4

Tossed Italian Salad

Chopped romaine hearts
Grape tomatoes
Cucumbers
Carrots
1-2 tablespoons of Chef Kevin's salad dressing (or olive oil and vinegar to taste)

Apple Balsamic Vinaigrette

1 apple, peeled and cored
1/3 cup of balsamic vinegar
2/3 cup of canola oil
Pinch of rosemary, fresh or dried
Pinch of dry mustard

Place all the ingredients in a blender and blend at high speed for one minute. Remove from blender and strain through a fine strainer.

Note: you can substitute any firm fruit to serve as the base of this dressing. For example, try experimenting with pears, plums, or peaches.

Serves 4

Roasted Shallot Vinaigrette

3 French shallots, peeled, tossed lightly in olive oil, and roasted at 375° for 20 minutes
1/3 cup balsamic vinegar
2/3 cup extra virgin olive oil
1/4 teaspoon dry mustard
Pinch of fresh or dry thyme
1 garlic clove, peeled
Salt and pepper for seasoning

Place all the ingredients except the salt and pepper in a blender and blend at a high speed until the mixture takes a milky consistency. Remove from the blender and season with salt and pepper.

Serves 4

Lemon Parmesan Dressing

1/3 cup fresh squeezed lemon juice
2/3 cup extra virgin olive oil
1/3 cup grated Parmesan (or any other hard cheese)
2 celery stalks
4 pink peppercorns
1 teaspoon Dijon mustard

Place all the ingredients except the salt in a blender and blend at a high speed for 1 minute. Remove and strain. Season with the salt.

Serves 4

Salt Substitute

2 tablespoons of:
Cayenne pepper
Dried garlic powder
Dried onion powder
Dried thyme
Dried oregano
Dried basil
Dried parsley flakes
Dried pink peppercorns
Dried savory
Dried black pepper
Dried lemon peel
1/2 teaspoon dried ground nutmeg
3 tablespoons dried marjoram

Mix all the ingredients in a bowl. With a spice grinder, finely blend all the ingredients. Remix in a separate bowl. Save in an airtight container and use as you would use salt.

★ Strawberry Yogurt Pudding
★
★ ★

1 envelope of unflavored gelatin
1/2 cup of boiling water
2 tablespoons of honey
1 teaspoon of orange extract
1 cup of plain low-fat yogurt
1/2 cup of pureed strawberries
2 tablespoons of graham cracker crumbs

Dissolve gelatin thoroughly in boiling water. Mix in honey. Add remaining ingredients except for the graham cracker crumbs. Divide among 4 dessert dishes, sprinkle each one with graham cracker crumbs and chill.

Serves 4

Fresh Fruit with Honey Vanilla Yogurt

2 cups of plain yogurt
2 tablespoons of good honey
1/2 teaspoon of pure vanilla extract
1/2 pint of fresh blueberries
1/2 pint of fresh raspberries
1 pint of fresh strawberries, cut in half

Combine the yogurt, honey, and vanilla extract and mix the berries together. Spoon the fruit into serving bowls and top with the yogurt.

Serves 4

Pears Poached in Dark Grape Juice

6 pears
2 tablespoons lemon juice
2 cups of dark grape juice
2 cups of blackcurrant juice
2 tablespoons of sweet sherry
4 cloves
1 cup of low-fat natural yogurt
1/2 teaspoon ground cinnamon
1 tablespoon honey

Core and peel the pears, placing them into a bowl filled with cold water and lemon juice, to prevent them from browning. Put the grape and blackcurrant juice, sherry, and cloves in a large saucepan and add the pears. Bring the liquid to a boil, and then reduce to a simmer. Cover and cook for 30-40 minutes, or until the pears are tender. Remove from the heat and leave the pears to cool in the syrup. Remove the pears from the syrup. Strain the syrup into a pan, bring to a boil, then reduce the heat and simmer for 40 minutes or until reduced by about two-thirds.

To serve, place one pear on each serving dish, cool the syrup slightly, and pour over the pears. Just before serving, thoroughly mix the yogurt, cinnamon, and honey together and spoon over the pears.

Serves 4

★ Slim Pastry Cream
★ ★

> 1/2 envelope of unflavored gelatin
> 1/2 cup of cold water
> 1 cup of skim milk
> 1 tablespoon of cornstarch
> 2 omega-3 egg yolks
> 3 tablespoons of honey
> 1 teaspoon of vanilla extract

In a small saucepan, sprinkle gelatin over cold water. Set aside for two minutes, to soften. In a medium size saucepan, heat 3/4 cup of the skim milk. Shake the remaining milk and cornstarch in a jar with a tight-fitting lid, or whisk together until well blended. In a small bowl, beat egg yolks and honey together until lemon colored. Beat in cornstarch mixture. Pour hot skim milk into the top of a double boiler and set over hot water. Slowly whisk in egg yolk mixture and cook, stirring constantly until custard coats the back of a wooden spoon. Remove from heat and pour into a medium size bowl. Heat softened gelatin until dissolved. Stir into pastry cream, mix in the vanilla, and allow to cool before serving.

Serves 4

Cottage Cheese Pie

1/2 tablespoon Smart Balance or alternative trans fat-free spread
3 tablespoons graham cracker crumbs
1/4 teaspoon ground cinnamon
16 ounces of low-fat cream-style cottage cheese
4 teaspoons of cornstarch
1/4 cup of honey
1 1/2 teaspoons freshly squeezed lemon juice
2 omega-3 eggs
10 fresh strawberries, halved

Preheat oven to 350 degrees. Rinse an 8 1/2 inch pie plate in hot water. Dry well and rub Smart Balance on bottom of pie plate (using all the spred). Sprinkle pie plate with graham cracker crumbs and press lightly to make crust.

Put remaining ingredients, except strawberries, into a food processor and blend until smooth. Pour over crust and bake on middle shelf of the oven until set, about 30 minutes. Cool well, then garnish with strawberry halves.

10 servings

★ Raspberry Cheese Pie

3 cups of fresh raspberries
1/4 cup of cornstarch
1/2 cup of honey warmed
1 pound low-fat cottage cheese
2 omega-3 eggs
2 tablespoons of honey
1 1/2 teaspoons of vanilla extract

Preheat oven to 350 degrees. Toss raspberries and cornstarch together in a medium size bowl, breaking some berries with a fork to release the juice. Add warmed honey, mix well, and turn into prepared pie plate. Bake on middle shelf of the oven for 20 minutes.

While raspberries are baking, combine the cottage cheese, eggs, honey, and vanilla extract in a food processor and blend until smooth. Pour over the raspberries and return the plate to the oven. Reduce heat to 300 degrees and bake another 30 minutes. Allow to cool before serving.

Serves 4-6

Chocolate Mousse

2 tablespoons of cocoa
2 leaves of sheet gelatin
10 ounces of silken tofu
1 tablespoon of brandy
2 egg whites
1/4 cup of caster sugar

Stir the cocoa with 1/4 cup of hot water until dissolved. In a separate small bowl, cover the leaf gelatin with cold water and allow to sit until the leaves become soft. When this happens, drain off all the excess cold water and return the leaves to the bowl. In a separate small pan, bring some water to a boil. Sit the bowl with the gelatin over the hot water and stir until the gelatin dissolves.

Drain the tofu and place in blender. Add the cocoa mixture and brandy and blend until smooth, scraping down the sides. Transfer this mixture to a bowl. Whisk the egg whites in a clean dry bowl, until soft peaks form. Gradually add the sugar, beating well between each addition, until stiff and glossy peaks form. Fold into the chocolate mixture, and then add the melted gelatin mixture, ensuring that you mix well. Divide into 4 dishes. Refrigerate for several hours, or until set.

Serves 4

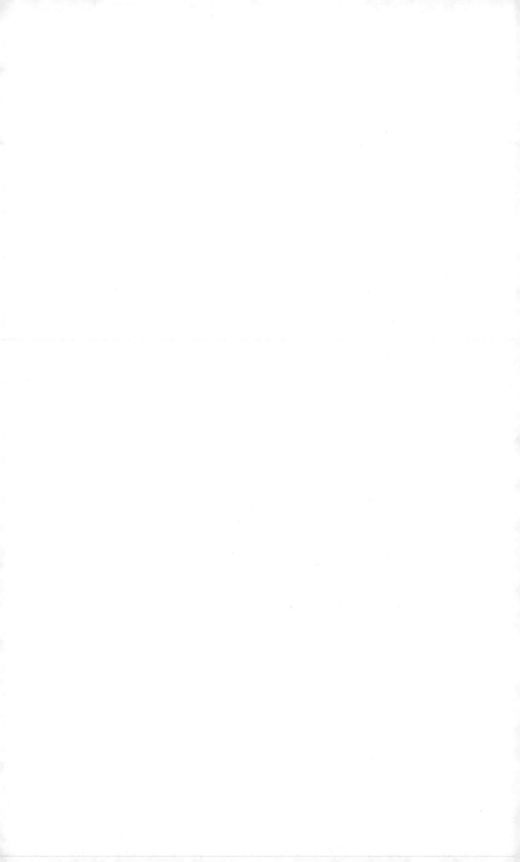

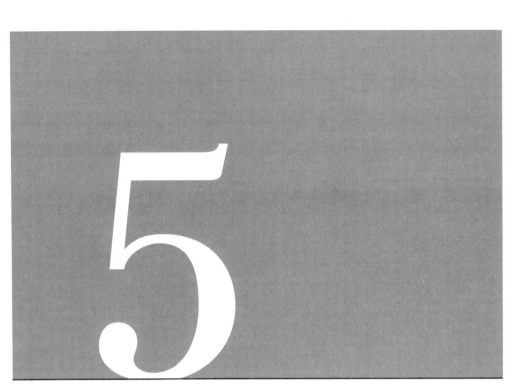

Part 5
Appendix

DETERMINING YOUR BODY MASS INDEX (BMI) AND DISEASE RISK

Body mass index, or BMI, is the most reliable measure of body weight as it relates to your health and wellness. BMI considers a person's weight in relation to his or her height and is calculated by dividing weight in kilograms by height in meters squared (BMI = kg/m^2).

A BMI of 18 to 24 is considered normal or ideal. A BMI of 25 to 29 is considered overweight, and a BMI of 30 or above obese. Waist size also affects your risk of disease. Refer to the charts on the next page to establish your BMI and assess your disease risk.

To use the table to the right, find the appropriate height (in inches) in the left-hand column. Move across the row to find your weight. The number at the top of the column is the BMI for your height and weight.

BMI	19	20	21	22	23	24	25	26	27	28	29	30	31	32
Height (in)														
58	91	96	100	105	110	115	119	124	129	134	138	143	167	191
59	94	99	104	109	114	119	124	128	133	138	143	148	173	198
60	97	102	107	112	118	123	128	133	138	143	148	153	179	204
61	100	106	111	116	122	127	132	137	143	148	153	158	185	211
62	104	109	115	120	126	131	136	142	147	153	158	164	191	218
63	107	113	118	124	130	135	141	146	152	158	163	169	197	225
64	110	116	122	128	134	140	145	151	157	163	169	174	204	232
65	114	120	126	132	138	144	150	156	162	168	174	180	210	240
66	118	124	130	136	142	148	155	161	167	173	179	186	216	247
67	121	127	134	140	146	153	159	166	172	178	185	191	223	255
68	125	131	138	144	151	158	164	171	177	184	190	197	230	262
69	128	135	142	149	155	162	169	176	182	189	196	203	236	270
70	132	139	146	153	160	167	174	181	188	195	202	207	243	278
71	136	143	150	157	165	172	179	186	193	200	208	215	250	286
72	140	147	154	162	169	177	184	191	199	206	213	221	258	294
73	144	151	159	166	174	182	189	197	204	212	219	227	265	302
74	148	155	163	171	179	186	194	202	210	218	225	233	272	311
75	152	160	168	176	184	192	200	208	216	224	232	240	279	319
76	156	164	172	180	189	197	205	213	221	230	238	246	287	328

Risk of Associated Disease According to BMI and Waist Size

BMI		Waist less than or equal to 40 in. (men) or 35 in. (women)	Waist greater than or equal to 40 in. (men) or 35 in. (women)
18.5 or less	Underweight	--	N/A
18.5-24.9	Normal	--	N/A
25.0-29.9	Overweight	Increased	Increased
30.0-34.9	Obese	High	High
35.0-39.9	Obese	Very High	Very High
40 or greater	Extremely Obese	Extremely High	Extremely High

INDEX

Italicized references indicate recipes.

American Heart Association, 76, 98, 181, 184, 186
  "Heart Healthy Diet", 184
American Institute of Cancer Research, 42, 165
American Journal of Clinical Nutrition, 30, 34, 52
American Journal of Epidemiology, 63, 98
American Medical Association, 204
Amino acids, 91
  arginine, 91
  homocysteine, 182
Amount of food in a serving. *See* Serving size
Anabolic storage hormone, 15
Animal protein, 43, 60, 61, 65, 69
  vs. vegetable protein, 58, 184, 187, 198
  See also Dairy products, Meat, Soy
Annals of Internal Medicine, 63, 70
Annual Conference on Cardiovascular Prevention (43rd), 98
Anthocyanins, 48, 49, 55
Anti-inflammatory benefits, 47, 55, 198, 201
  of aspirin, 193
  vitamin E, 202
Antioxidants, 47, 48, 207–08
  anthocyanins, 48, 49, 55
  and disease prevention, 139, 167, 171, 180, 183, 187, 191, 198, 202
  flavonoids, 27-28, 52, 54, 137-38, 139, 149, 183
  lycopene, 48–49, 174
  phytochemicals, 27, 47-50, 53-54, 90, 168, 183
  in red wine, 36–37, 137, 149
  squalene, 158-59, 167, 170, 176
  sulforaphane, 49-50, 110
  and tea, 37-38, 137, 168
  and vitamins C and E, 90, 92, 202, 205, 206
Antioxidant score, 55
Apple Balsamic Vinaigrette, *255*
Apples, 53, 111, 179, 187, 193,198, 202
  Pork Tenderloin with Apples and Dried Apricots, *235*
  Medallions of Veal with Celeriac and Apples, *236*
  Apple Balsamic Vinaigrette, *255*
  See also Fruits
Apricots, dried, 157, 210, 211
  Benefits of, 53, 56, 99, 111, 179, 190
  Cantaloupe with Lime Juice and Dried Apricots, *216*

Salsa, *215*
sample menus, 210–11
Sautéed Spinach with Poached Eggs, *217*
Scrambled Omega-3 Eggs with Salsa, *215*
Smoked Salmon Frittata, *219*
Warm Breakfast Salad, *219*
Breast cancer, 61, 71, 167, 169–72
monthly self-examination, 172
recommended supplements, 171
See also Cancer
British Dental Journal, 35
British Medical Journal, 78
Broccoli, 17, 46, 48, 49–50, 110, 111, 133, 153
Broccoli Florets with Lemon Manchego Cheese, 222
and disease, 166, 170, 179, 180, 183, 187, 190, 193, 198, 202
BroccoSprouts, 110, 111
Broiled Chicken Breast with Cashews and Cauliflower, *227*
Brussels Sprouts, 48, 50, 111
and disease, 166, 170, 179, 187, 193, 198, 202
Roasted Brussels Sprouts and Shallots, *251*
Butter, 79, 115, 119, 155, 158, 182, 194
substitutes for, 155, 187

C
Cabbage (Oriental) Salad, *249*
Caffeine, 156
and high blood pressure, 191
Calcium, 76, 139, 176, 190, 194, 195, 207
leaching of
and diet sodas, 34–35, 155–56
excessive protein, 63
and magnesium, 207
and osteoarthritis, 198
Cancer, 23–24, 27, 37, 60, 192–95
and phytochemicals, 48-50
prevention of, 164–76
breast cancer, 169–72
colon cancer, 192–95
prostate cancer, 173–76
recommended supplements, 168
Cancer Causes and Control, 175
Canned goods, 118, 147, 151
list of good and bad choices, 118

Canola oil, 121, 159
  See also Monounsaturated fats
Cantaloupe with Lime Juice and Dried Apricots, *216*
Carcinogens, 49, 61, 134, 166, 167
Cardiotoxic emotions, 184, 191
Cardiovascular benefits of omega 3, 76
Cardiovascular disease, 22, 76
  risk factor, 181–183
  See also Heart disease
Carnivorous fish. *See* Seafood
Carrots, 17, 18, 47, 111
  and disease, 166, 170, 193
  Spinach Salad with Almonds and Shredded Carrots, *229*
Catechin, 168
Cauliflower, 48, 111
  and disease, 166, 170, 193
  Broiled Chicken Beast with Cashews and Cauliflower, *227*
  Roasted Cauliflower, *250*
Center for Science in the Public Interest, 72
Centers for Disease Control, 162
Cereals, 116, 117
Cheese, 43, 115
  Avocado and Tomato Salad with Feta Cheese, *224*
  Baby Spinach, Feta, Pine Nuts and Strawberry Salad, *252*
  Breakfast Salad with Ricotta Cheese, *218*
  Broccoli Florets with Lemon Manchego Cheese, *222*
  Cottage Cheese Pie, *261*
  health concerns, 65, 79, 176
  healthy snacks, 99
  Omega-3 Eggs Veggie Omelet, *219*
  Quick Homemade Veggie Pizza, *223*
  Raspberry Cheese Pie, *262*
  Roast Beef and Swiss Pita Sandwich, *229*
  Roasted Shallot Vinaigrette Dressing, *256*
  yogurt cheese, 64, 138, 158
Chef Kevin. *See* Graham, Kevin (Chef)
Chef Kevin's Vegetable Juice, *218*
Chicken. *See* Poultry and game
Chocolate, 125, 148, 149
Chocolate Mousse, *263*
Cholesterol, 20, 22, 69, 71, 73, 74, 151–52, 185–88
Chondroitin, 199
Chromium, 180

Eggs, 115, 146
   and cholesterol, 151–52
   frittatas
      Egg White Frittata with Bell Peppers, *214*
      Smoked Salmon Frittata, *219*
   omega-3 eggs, 59, 65, 80, 115, 135, 152
      Scrambled Omega-3 eggs with Salsa, *215*
   omelets
      Caramelized Onion Omelet, *213*
      Omega-3 Eggs Veggie Omelet, *219*
   Sautéed Spinach with Poached Eggs, *217*
Eicosanoids, 61, 67, 74–75
Emotions, cardiotoxic, 184, 191
Endorphins, 130
Enzymes, 29, 50
   phase 2 enzymes, 49
EPA. *See* Omega-3 fatty acids
Exercise, 81–88, 106, 157
   amount and kind, 89
   and disease, 166, 170, 175, 177, 182, 187, 190, 193-94, 197, 201
   motivation, 88
Expeller pressed canola oil. *See* Canola oil

F

Farm raised salmon. *See* Seafood
Fast food restaurants
   strategies for, 143–44
Fat cells, 15
FDA, 58, 72-73
Fiber, 26-30, 91, 186
Fish. *See* Seafood
Fish oils, 147, 152, 156, 206
   as source of omega 3, 77
Flavonoids, 27, 54, 137, 139, 149, 183
Flaxseed oil vs. fish oils, 152
Folic acid, 67, 171, 182, 205
Food, Nutrition and the Prevention of Cancer: A Global Perspective,
  165
Food & Wine, 209
Food labels, 107–09
   ingredients to avoid, 108
Free radicals, 48, 135, 201
Fresh Blended Tomato, *214*

J

JAMA. See Journal of the American Medical Association
Johns Hopkins University, 70
Joint-health supplements, 198–99
Joseph, James, 53
Journal of Agriculture and Food Chemistry, 27, 149
Journal of Clinical Endocrinology and Metabolism, 35–36
Journal of the American Medical Association, 23, 41, 93
Journal of the National Cancer Institute, 24, 174, 195
Juices, 38, 129
    Chef Kevin's Vegetable Juice, *218*

K

Kale, 48, 50, 111, 153
    and disease, 166, 170, 187, 190, 198, 202,
    Braised Kale, *251*

L

Labels. *See* Food labels
Lamb. *See* Meats
LDL
    elevated by trans fats, 71
    and insulin resistance syndrome, 20
    and iron intake, 188
    lowering, 73, 185–88
    and nuts, 93
    recommended levels, 186
    and saturated fats, 69
    and soy products, 60
Legumes, 27-28, 29, 32, 59, 65, 120, 124, 139-140
    and disease, 179, 183, 190
    See also Beans
Lemon Parmesan Dressing, *256*
Lentils, 16-17, 27-28, 29, 32, 58-59, 124, 254
    and disease, 179, 194–95
    with Salmon Cubes, *226*
    See also Beans, Legumes
Liquid calories, 33–38, 105
    list of good choices, 39
Loma Linda University, 93
Louisiana State University, 34
Low-carb diets, 12–13, 26

Baby Spinach, Feta, Pine Nuts and Strawberry Salad, *252*
Broiled Chicken Breast with Cashews and Cauliflower, *227*
Granola, *213*
and disease, 168, 171, 176, 183, 187, 195, 202
list of good and bad choices, 92, 95, 120
preparation, 136–37
size of servings, 92, 95
Spinach salad with Almonds and Shredded Carrots, *229*
NWCR. *See* National Weight Control Registry

O

Oatmeal, 30, 117, 210
Almond Oatmeal Pancakes, *216*
Boneless Skinless Trout in Oatmeal, *242*
Oats, 30, 32, 117, 122, 153
and disease, 179, 186
Homemade Granola, *213*
Obesity
and diabetes, 177
and osteoarthritis, 196
and TV watching, 87
Oils, 43, 121, 135–36
See also Monounsaturated fats, Polyunsaturated fats
Olive oil, 73, 79, 121, 131, 135, 143
extra virgin, 153,158–59, 191
and disease, 167, 170, 175–76, 179, 182, 184, 187–88, 194
See also Monounsaturated fats, Oils
Omega-3 eggs, 59, 65, 80, 133, 135, 151–52
and disease, 179–80, 182, 194, 197
Omega-3 Eggs Veggie Omelet, *219*
Scrambled Omega-3 Eggs with Salsa, *215*
Omega-3 fatty acids, 58-59, 61, 76–78, 80, 106, 206
eggs. *See* Omega-3 eggs
and disease, 167, 170, 175, 179, 182, 194, 197, 200–01
relationship to omega 6, 74–76, 92, 150
sources of, 60, 90, 92, 112, 115, 152
Omega-6 fatty acids, 61
and disease, 167, 170, 175, 197, 202
relationship to omega-3, 74–76, 92, 150
Omelets. *See* Eggs
Onions, 48, 51, 110-11, 133-34, 151, 153
Caramelized Onion Omelet, *213*

Soy, 59, 60, 99, 115, 126, 130, 139, 158
 and disease, 170–171, 173, 175, 179–180, 182, 184, 187–188, 194, 197
 Tempeh/Veggie Wrap, *225*
 vs. animal protein, 60
Soy milk, 39, 59, 65, 79, 99, 115, 133, 135, 148, 158
 and disease, 176, 190
Soybeans, 17, 27, 32, 77, 121, 124, 139, 158
 and disease, 167, 190, 195, 197, 202
Spices, 130, 134, 139, 198
Spinach, 48, 56, 80, 111, 134, 153, 166
 Baby Spinach, Feta, Pine Nuts, and Strawberry Salad, *252*
 and disease, 170, 187, 190, 193, 198, 202
 Sautéed Spinach with Poached Eggs, *217*
 Spinach Salad with Almonds and Shredded Carrots, *229*
Splenda, 153–54, 212
Squalene, 158–59, 167, 170, 176
 See also Antioxidants
Stomach capacity, 44
Strawberries, 17, 53, 55, 56
 Baby Spinach, Feta, Pine Nuts and Strawberry Salad, *252*
 and disease, 183, 187, 190
 Strawberry Yogurt Pudding, *258*
Strength building activities and exercise, 89
Stretching activities and exercise, 89
Sulforaphane, 49
Supplements, 156, 204–08
 and disease, 168, 171, 176, 180, 182, 183, 188, 195, 198–99, 203
Sweeteners, dietetic, 153–54

T
Tappenade, *241*
Tea, 37–38, 39, 129, 137, 168, 191, 199, 210
 green tea, 54, 149, 187–88
Television and exercise, 87
Tempeh/Veggie Wrap, *225*
Tobacco, 168
Tofu, 59, 115, 139
 Chocolate Mousse, *236*
 and disease, 171, 175, 180, 187, 190
 tofu in Miso Sauce, *239*
 See also Soy

V

W

Waffles, whole grain (frozen), 119
Waist size
   and insulin resistance syndrome, 20
   and risk of associated disease, 268
Walking, 85
   See also Exercise
Warm Breakfast Salad, *219*
Water, 35–36
   recommended amount, 39
Watercress and Romaine Lettuce with Cucumber Dressing, *225*
Watermelon, 16, 18, 175
Weight loss
   amount to expect, 145
   and exercise, 81–88
   lack of, 146
Weisburger, John, 37
"Western diet", 23
Wild salmon, 65, 112, 136, 150–51
   See also Salmon, seafood
Wine, red. *See* Red wine

Y

Yogurt, 43, 62, 65, 79, 114, 115, 133, 148,
   and disease, 190, 194
   as mayonnaise substitute, 138, 157
   Fresh Fruits with Honey Vanilla Yogurt, 259
   Strawberry Yogurt Pudding, 258
   See also Yogurt cheese
Yogurt cheese, 64, 138, 157–58